WHOM THE GODS LOVE DIE YOUNG

*A Modern Medical Perspective on Illnesses
That Caused the Early Death of Famous People*

by

Roy Macbeth Pitkin, M.D.

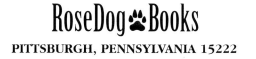

RoseDog✹Books

PITTSBURGH, PENNSYLVANIA 15222

For more information or to order additional books,
please contact:
RoseDog Books
701 Smithfield Street
Third Floor
Pittsburgh, Pennsylvania 15222
U.S.A.
1-800-834-1803
www.rosedogbookstore.com

To

MARCIA

My staunchest supporter, most helpful critic, and best friend

CONTENTS

PREFACE

THIS COLLECTION OF ESSAYS CONCERNS MEDICAL HISTORY, SPECIFICALLY the history of certain selected diseases and how they have evolved over the past century or two with respect to their frequency, diagnosis and treatment, and physicians' understanding of their nature. To introduce each disease, I have invoked a well-known historical figure who died of the condition before the age of 40. Thus, this book is about what might be termed "early adult mortality." Its main title comes from Lord Byron (Don Juan, Canto IV, Stanza 12) who himself died at 36.

The book begins with an introductory chapter, which reviews historical trends in mortality and its causes, defines life expectancy and other relevant terms, and glimpses into the future of early adult mortality. Ten chapters then follow, one devoted to each historical figure (in chronological order) and his or her cause of death. I divided these chapters into three sections of approximately equal length: first a brief biography, a summary of why the person is well-known; then a description, in as much detail as the information available permits, of his or her health, illness, and death; and finally a modern medical perspective on that illness, concluding with a speculation as to the outcome if the subject had the particular disease today.

In choosing the historical figures and diseases to cover, I found particularly useful as a first step the remarkable book by Norman and Betty Donaldson entitled *How Did They Die?* Published first in a single volume in 1983 and then re-published with additions in three volumes in the early 1990s (by St. Martin's Press, New York), it consists of short vignettes about the last days and last words of famous figures throughout history. The Donaldson book allowed me to screen for those well-known people who died of natural causes before age 40, and from this screen I then selected those persons, and especially those diseases, that seemed particularly interesting. In most but not all cases, the diseases chosen have changed remarkably with respect to incidence, diagnosis, or outcome since the historical figure died of them. To learn about the subjects I chose to introduce each topic, I read two to four full-length biographies of each. In several cases, physicians interested in literature or art or history had published analyses of the person's health, illness, and death, and these proved especially useful. To inform myself about history and current status of the various diseases, I consulted medical texts, articles in medical journals, and web sites. In addition, having graduated from medical school in 1959, I brought my personal knowledge and perspectives accumulated over 50 years as a physician to bear.

Decisions about referencing the sources proved especially difficult. On the one hand, my scientific background argued for full documentation of each point. On the other, I recognize that most readers find repetitive footnotes and other text references distracting. In the end, I decided against citing references in the text, choosing instead to list the sources I consulted at the end of each chapter. Everything within a chapter, save for information from my personal knowledge or experience, came from the sources listed.

Many colleagues, friends, and family members helped in various ways in the writing of this book. Several staff members of the American College of Obstetricians and Gynecologists (ACOG) gave invaluable assistance. Rebecca D. Rinehart, Director of Publications for ACOG, provided invaluable advice—as she has many other times over the years—in negotiating the complex and often arcane ways of publishing. Cindy Woo of her staff identified several important illustrations. Debra Scarborough, Archivist of ACOG's Resource Center, was extremely helpful in tracking down several older references and statistical data. Bill Pitkin constructed the graphs (using data I provided him from various sources) that appear in three chapters. Bob Dolfi and Damon Lanza of *Lanza Legend* generously provided important data, not available elsewhere, relating to Mario Lanza, along with an unpublished photograph. Many others contributed photographs and, where appropriate, I have indicated the source in the legends to individual illustrations.

I am especially indebted to Richard M. Freeman, long time friend and colleague, for his original idea of a book about famous people who died young and for his valuable reviews of several of the chapters. Steve Derose provided helpful medical review of several chapters. A number of friends and neighbors read individual chapters and contributed helpful suggestions; particularly noteworthy in this regard are Donald Robertson and John Walsh who reviewed every chapter (along with patiently trying to improve my tennis game). My wife, Marcia J. Pitkin, scrutinized the full manuscript with her customary eagle eye.

Roy Macbeth Pitkin
La Quinta, California
May 2008

CHAPTER 1

INTRODUCTION

THE ORIGINS OF MODERN SCIENTIFIC MEDICINE CAN BE TRACED TO THE late 19th century when, spurred by a number of discoveries and inventions, fundamental concepts of the nature of disease began to change radically. For hundreds of years before that time, disease was regarded generally as reflecting a disturbance in the body's equilibrium and the overall therapeutic goal was to restore proper balance. Many illnesses were thought to be due to imbalances induced by toxins, leading to widespread use of such treatments as purging, bloodletting, and blistering to rid the body of these presumably noxious substances.

It is easy, perhaps too easy, to fault, for example, George Washington's physicians for their relentless bloodletting in treatment of his throat infection, something we now realize did nothing for the problem and quite likely hastened the death of this American hero. As misguided as this therapy seems to the modern eye, it was consistent with the teaching of medical authorities of that time. Further, physicians of the pre-modern era lacked many of the critical adjuncts to diagnosis that would come later; for example, the stethoscope was invented in 1819, the clinical thermometer in 1870, and the blood pressure cuff not until 1901. Finally, even if early physicians had possessed the knowledge, understanding, and diagnostic aids that would come later, effective drugs were virtually non-existent. The therapeutic options were extremely limited and most of the popular pharmaceuticals owed their favored status to an ability to cause easily recognized effects. Agents such as camphor, mercury, and ergot were used widely and for a variety of different conditions, and of course the most popular of all was opium. Opium and later one of its active components, morphine, caused effects (relief of pain and a sense of well being) that were easily recognized as well as pleasant. Opium in its various forms was part of nearly every prescribed therapy and also found its way into many patent medicines sold over the counter.

1

Medicine began to change during the last several decades of the 19th century as the theory of disease moved away from emphasis on "internal balance" to broader concepts of how different types of illnesses manifest themselves and how they interfered with normal functioning in specific ways. A major force driving this change came from the German school, led chiefly by Rudolf Virchow, with its emphasis on careful postmortem examination and then relating the findings systematically to the decedent's clinical history and physical characteristics. There is probably no better example of how the understanding of the nature of disease changed than the case of infections. Certain diseases had long been suspected time of being transmitted from person to person and, indeed, the microscope had been invented in the early 1600s. Nevertheless, it was not until the last third of the 19th century that Pasteur in France and Koch in Germany made their seminal observations that laid the foundations of the germ theory of disease.

Concomitant with the scientific advances in medicine came increasing professionalism. Medical schools moved from being short-term diploma mills toward true academic units with curricula that emphasized the disciplined, scientific approach to diagnosis and treatment. Physicians formed themselves into professional societies that, among other initiatives, lobbied for laws establishing licensing procedures.

VITAL STATISTICS

The term "vital statistics" refers to data collected, tabulated, and analyzed by governmental bodies from registration of various life events such as births, deaths, marriages, and divorces. Although health statistics began to be gathered in the late 18th century, it wasn't until the dawn of the 20th century that registration of these events became routine and eventually mandatory, and then only in developed nations such as the United States and Western European countries. The century just past could justifiably be termed the "statistical century" and government at all levels has come to rely increasingly on such data in planning public health programs to meet its population's needs and obligations. Moreover, the general public has become increasingly knowledgeable about health statistics and interested in their implications.

Life Expectancy

One of the health statistics of greatest interest is that of "life expectancy," the average length of time members of a population will live. It is generally recognized that average length of life, at least in the United States, differs by gender (with females outliving males by two or three years) and race

(with whites outliving other races by four or five years), and data are tabulated both overall and with respect to these differences. Much fanfare
accompanied the recent announcement that overall average life expectancy
from birth in the United States, which had been increasing progressively
since first tabulated, appeared to cross 80 years for the first time in 2005.

For most of history, the life of humans has been, in the famous words of the
17th century philosopher Thomas Hobbes, "solitary, poor, nasty, brutish,
and short." The average life expectancy of an infant born during Roman
times is estimated to have been 25 years. There was minimal improvement
for nearly 2000 years; even as late as 1850, the corresponding value in the
United States was only about 35.

Although most people are aware that life expectancy has increased dramatically over the last century or so, the concept involves nuances and caveats
that are probably appreciated and understood fully by relatively few. Average
life expectancy from birth in the United States has gone from 47.3 years in
1900-1902 to 77.3 in 2002. As noted earlier, pre-1900 figures are incomplete, but available information suggests an overall average of 40 years in
about 1870. Thus, in view of the provisional figure of 80 years in 2005
announced recently, it would seem at first glance that people in the United
States now live twice as long as they did a century and a third ago. But it is
not quite so simple, mainly because the value depends directly on the starting age of the group under consideration. Most commonly, the term life
expectancy refers to the time <u>from birth</u> (i.e., average lifetime anticipated for
a baby born in the specific year). Thus, it represents an estimate of what will
happen in the future, and it may therefore be modified by unexpected
changes in population health. Moreover and more importantly, as an average, it is influenced most by data at the extremes, in this case deaths during
childhood.

Deaths in infancy and childhood, extremely common until about the middle of the 20th century, have diminished remarkably since then. Many reasons for the decline can be posited: improved sanitation and better living
conditions; better nutrition, immunizations against childhood infections,
and antibiotics. The phenomenal drop in infant and childhood mortality is
nowhere more evident than in the increased life expectancy since birth.
However, the change in life expectancy at later ages is much less dramatic, a
difference illustrated in this figure in which life expectancy at birth and at
age 10 years (when most childhood deaths would have occurred) are portrayed graphically. Over the 20th century, the increase in life expectancy at
age 10 was scarcely half that of life expectancy at birth (33% vs. 63%).

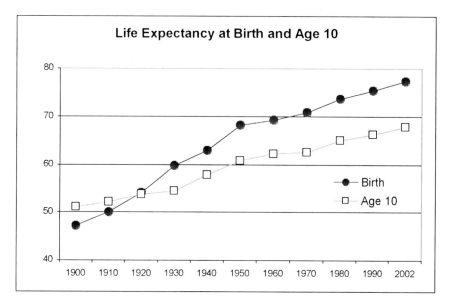

Causes of Death

Before the advent of scientific medicine, as knowledge and understanding of disease processes remained primitive, diagnosis was anything but accurate. As noted previously, concepts of disease were primitive and diagnostic labels often vague. Even when a specific disease was recognized, there was controversy as to its nature. For example, consumption (which we now call tuberculosis) was extremely common but there were violent disagreements among medical authorities, continuing until the mid- to late 19th century, as to whether it was contagious or hereditary. Further, many of the diagnostic labels applied to illnesses were vague and lacking in meaning, at least from today's perspective.

In the United States and most other developed nations, a "death certificate" must be completed by a licensed physician whenever a person dies. This certificate must identify the presumed cause(s) of death in reasonably specific terms (e.g., vague or general terms such as "old age" are not permitted). Information from the death certificate, collected and tabulated by public health authorities, forms the basis of the mortality trends reviewed throughout this book as evidence of changing disease frequency and outcome.

In reality, even today the cause(s) of death listed on the death certificate are often less than certain, and typically they represent the attending physician's "best guess." The actual cause of death can be determined with greater certainty by autopsy (i.e., postmortem dissection and examination) but this procedure is only mandated in instances in which foul play is possible or other legal issue exists. However, even in cases where autopsy is not required legally, it has long been regarded as crucial to the advancement of medical education and research. As noted previously, the modern era of medicine actually began with the systematic correlation between autopsy findings and clinical history.

Until relatively recently, autopsy was at the heart of scientific medicine, offering improved understanding of disease and better methods of diagnosis and treatment. In the 1960s, the rate of autopsy of hospital deaths in the United States and Western Europe was around 60%, and even higher in teaching hospitals where it was considered a marker of quality of the academic program. Authorities regarded autopsies as essential in recognizing inaccuracies in clinical diagnosis and thereby advancing medical knowledge, as well as in providing specific and definite information to a decedent's family.

Over the last 30 or 40 years, autopsy rates have fallen markedly. Presently, the rate is only about 10% of all deaths in hospitals, and undoubtedly even lower in non-teaching hospitals. The usual explanation for this change is that modern methods of diagnosis, especially imaging techniques, are so accurate that uncertainty in clinical diagnosis and discrepancy between clinical and autopsy diagnosis have both become rare. Another consideration, seldom mentioned but certainly a factor, is the dilemma of financial coverage of autopsies. Previously, the autopsy was considered part of a hospital's cost of doing business, but rising concerns about overall costs of health care have led to scrutiny of all budgetary aspects. Health financing organizations such as insurance carriers are reluctant to assume autopsy costs and, surely, a decedent's family and friends cannot to be expected to pay them. Thus, cost is undoubtedly an important factor in the declining autopsy rate. Many medical authorities have expressed concerns about the impending disappearance of the autopsy. Scientific studies indicate that inaccuracies in clinical diagnosis persist in spite of modern medical diagnostic measures, resulting in rates of discrepancy between clinical and autopsy diagnosis as high as 20-25%. For all these reasons, vital statistics based on death certificate information should not be regarded as infallible, although they represent the only source of population-based data.

THE FUTURE

What can we expect in the future appear with respect to early adult mortality? Quick perusal of the causes of death before the age of 40 reveals clear changes over the past 50 or 75 years. Until the early to mid-20th century, young adults who died usually died from "natural" causes, especially infectious diseases, but the last several decades have seen a declining frequency of these as causes of death. They have been replaced, largely though not entirely, with various "non-natural" conditions—accidents (especially vehicular accidents), suicide, homicide, and drug overdose. In the United States in 2002, accidents represented the leading cause of death of persons younger than 40 (in contrast, it was heart disease for those over 75 and cancer among 40-74 year-olds). Suicide and homicide are currently the fourth and fifth leading causes of death for individuals aged 10-60.

Of course, infections and other natural diseases have not disappeared. Moreover, there is some reason for concern that infectious diseases may become increasingly problematic. Antibiotic resistance is a significant threat, particularly with respect to global infections such as tuberculosis, but also in the case of more usual infections. Drugs have been developed that possess some activity against the human immunodeficiency virus (HIV) but none is curative and a vaccine to prevent HIV remains elusive. These concerns are important, but it still seems likely that early adult mortality in the future will pretty much mirror what we have seen in the recent past: mainly violent deaths due to accidents, suicide, homicide, and drug overdose.

One recent trend has caused great concern among public health authorities: what has been justifiably termed the "obesity epidemic." The marked increase in the frequency of excessive body weight has ominous implications extending across the entire population in developed countries, but its threat to those in the "prime of life" is especially alarming. Many different conditions, most of them potentially fatal, are linked to obesity:

- coronary heart disease
- high blood pressure
- high cholesterol and other lipids
- diabetes mellitus (type II)
- stroke
- gall bladder disease
- osteoarthritis
- sleep apnea
- some cancers (uterus, breast, colon)

Body weight is best expressed quantitatively by a value called body mass index (BMI) that takes into account height along with weight, calculated specifically by dividing weight in kilograms by the square of height in meters). BMI of 25-29.9 is considered overweight while a value of 30 or more defines obesity; some categorize BMI of 40 or more as "super obese."

The frequency of overweight and obesity in the population has increased in virtually all developed countries. The prevalence of obesity in American adults aged 20-74 more than doubled in the United States over a quarter century, from 15% in 1976-1980 to 32.9% in 2003-2004. Even greater increases occurred among children during the same interval; overweight went from 5% to 13.9% in ages 2-5, from 6.5% to 18.8% in ages 6-11, and from 5.1% to 17.4% in ages 12-19. This tripling of childhood overweight disorders, concerning by itself, becomes even more alarming when coupled with the appearance of medical disorders not seen previously in children. The most flagrant example is type II diabetes mellitus, formerly a disease exclusively of the elderly, but now being seen with increasingly in children who have become obese. Given its well-known predisposition to coronary and other vascular disease, it seems inevitable that a rash of heart attacks, stroke, kidney failure, and other similar conditions will be seen in the young adult population.

The ominous threat posed by obesity, especially childhood obesity, cannot be overstated. It threatens to arrest and even reverse the pervasive trend of steadily improving health outcomes so characteristic of the last century or two.

SOURCES

Porter R. *The Greatest Benefit to Mankind*: A Medical History of Humanity. Norton. New York and London. 1997

Hays JN. *The Burdens of Disease: Epidemics and Human Response in Western History*. Rutgers University Press. New Brunswick NJ. 1998

United States Life Tables, 2002. National Vital Statistics Reports, volume 53, number 6, November 10, 2004

Jemal A, Ward E, Hao Y, Thun. Trends in the leading causes of death in the United States, 1970-2002. *JAMA* 2005;294:1255-9

Shojania KG, Burton EC. The nonforensic autopsy. *New Engl J Med*; 2008: 873-5.

Roulson J, Benbow EW, Haselton PS. Discrepancies between clinical and autopsy diagnosis and the value of post mortem histology: a meta-analysis and review. *Histopathology* 2005;47:551-9

http://www.cdc.gov/nccdphh/dynpa/obesity. Accessed June 18, 2007.

CHAPTER 2

ROBERT BURNS AND RHEUMATIC HEART DISEASE

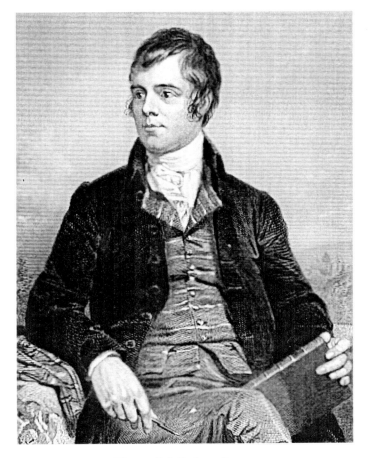

Figure 2.1 Robert Burns

IN SPITE OF A LIFE LASTING ONLY 37 YEARS AND SPENT IN GRINDING poverty in an out-of-the-way country, Robert Burns produced poems, lyrics, and letters that place him, in terms of both quality and quantity, among the world's best to ever put pen to paper. Raymond Bentman, Professor of English at Temple University, called him the first poet to address subjects that "have come to inspire and haunt the modern world: equality of all people; the delights and dangers of personal freedom outside the restraints of church and state; . . . the value of emotion; and the uncertainty of all knowledge." As a source of common expressions in modern English, Burns stands second only to Shakespeare. His lyrics gave emotion and meaning to traditional Scottish melodies and made them part of a worldwide heritage. Millions throughout the world sing *Auld Lang Syne* each New Year, though few probably know that Burns wrote the lyrics. Burns' early death probably resulted from a type of heart disease in which the heart valves have been damaged by previous rheumatic fever, a relatively common condition in the 18th century but one that medical therapy, particularly antibiotic treatment of streptococcal infections, along with improved living conditions, have made rare today.

Biography

In 18th-century Scotland, as in most of the world, wealth was concentrated in a very few hands, and almost all the population toiled dawn to dusk to eke out a wretched existence. Scotland may have had it worse than most countries, for its soil is poor and its climate marginal for agriculture. In addition, life had been made even more difficult by repressive measures imposed by the British government in response to the abortive attempt by Bonnie Prince Charlie and his followers to restore the Stuart monarchy in 1745-46.

It was this dismal set of circumstances that led William Burnes (or Burness—it is spelled both ways in different records) to leave his home in the Highlands in 1748, seeking better conditions in the south of the country. He obtained a position as a gardener to an aristocratic family, acquired a small plot of land in a village near Ayr, and built a house for himself and his new bride, Agnes Brown. As most houses that folks of Burnes' station lived in, this one had two rooms, one for the family and the other for the livestock. In this modest abode, by the light and heat of a peat fire, Agnes gave birth, on January 25, 1759, to a son they named Robert, after William's father. Agnes, a cheerful and lively woman, had a fine singing voice and knew traditional Scottish music. Robert's sensitivity and creativity can in all likelihood be traced to her; from his father came tenacity, a drive to learn, and a strong sense of responsibility. Six more children would follow over the years, and all would be involved in the hard work of the farm. It was a close-knit family and Robert always maintained the strong family ties of his childhood. He was especially close to his next-younger brother, Gilbert.

Although seriously disadvantaged by their country's rocky soil and inhospitable climate, Scots possessed one distinct advantage over citizens of other countries: the strong commitment to education that had characterized the Scottish ethic since the Protestant Reformation. Beginning a century before young Robert's birth, the Scots parliament passed legislation requiring each parish to see that all children in it were provided free education. The level of competence required was modest—ability to read and write at an elementary level and to make simple arithmetic calculations—and compliance was uneven, but this was by many years the first public education in the history of the world. William Burnes, though poor, was quite literate and well read, and he supplemented his children's public instruction by assigning them readings: the Bible, of course, but also Shakespeare, Milton, and Dryden. Additionally, he used some of his meager income to hire a tutor for his children. The periods of formal instruction were erratic, subject to interruption by urgent farm duties, but the Burnes children overall were educated to a level at or even above that of much more privileged families. In the case of young Robbie, it would yield benefits of a kind that could not be even dreamed-of.

In 1781, 22-year-old Robert went to Irvine to learn the trade of flax combing, which the family hoped would augment farming income. The flax venture, like so many others poor Scottish farmers tried, proved unsuccessful, but in Irvine Robert discovered the local library (another reflection of the Scottish commitment to education) and a bookstore, and his horizons exploded. He also discovered the "new" drink from the Highlands, whisky, and he experienced the first of what would eventually be many romantic encounters. After six months at Irvine, he had to return home because his father, as a result of crop failures and other misfortunes, was in financial difficulty. Moreover, William's health was deteriorating and, after a protracted illness, he died in February 1784. He and his eldest son were often at odds because of the latter's interest in music, dancing, and other activities Calvinist doctrine regarded as frivolous. Yet there were strong bonds between father and son, bonds that included respect and even a kind of affection. Later, in one of his most famous poems, *The Cotter's Saturday Night*, Robert would use his father as the inspiration for one of the main characters, the gentle patriarch.

Robert was now, at age 25, the head of the family and, in the weeks following his father's death, he took two actions. He changed the spelling of his last name to Burns and he and Gilbert took lease on a 100-acre farm called Mossgiel in the parish of Mauchline. Although Robert approached the new venture with enthusiasm and gave himself to it fully, in the end it led only to more backbreaking toil, crop failures, and ultimately financial ruin. After two years of discouragement, he gave up on Mossgiel and, at least for the time being, on farming.

When Robert began to write poetry is not known with certainty, but it almost surely was in his early teens. He later intimated that he formed ideas for poems or lyrics to traditional Scottish melodies while plowing or doing other farm work, and then wrote at night by candlelight. In any case, by the time of the ill-fated Mossgiel venture, he had accumulated enough writings, and more importantly was able to convince someone of their value, that his first volume of poetry was published. On July 31, 1786, John Wilson of Kilmarnock printed 600 copies of *Poems, Chiefly in the Scottish Dialect*. It was wildly successful, far beyond even the author's dreams, and it brought in money, which was duly plowed back into the losing farm operation. Encouraged by success in poetry and discouraged by failure in farming, Robert decided to go to Edinburgh.

The city that greeted Robert Burns on his arrival in November 1786 was considered the Athens of the North. It reflected such intellectual luminaries as the philosopher David Hume and the economist Adam Smith, both of whose writings were well known to Robert. All the powerful and wealthy of Scotland lived there and their salons and drawing rooms oozed elegance and culture. Burns' reputation had preceded him and all Edinburgh seemed anxious to see this "plowman poet." His poetry volume was reprinted, selling over 3000 copies, and he made a number of contacts with important people. He also took the opportunity to go on two extended tours, one to the Highlands and the other through the Lowlands, in the process learning his country's history and traditions.

The Edinburgh interlude was successful in producing some income from his writings, but Burns continued to be plagued by financial concerns. He once said his main hope was that his poetry would outlast his poverty. He gave serious consideration to immigrating to the West Indies, but ultimately he decided to remain in Scotland, hoping for some sort of position that would pay a steady wage. Through Edinburgh contacts he ultimately obtained a kind of civil service position as an excise man in Dumfries, about 50 miles south of the capital city. This position paid a steady stipend, but it was by no means a soft job. He had to travel around his assigned territory by horseback, often as much as 200 miles in a week, levying taxes on imports and local produce. However, his attraction to the soil remained still strong, so when he left Edinburgh after two years to take up his new position, he settled on a farm a few miles north of Dumfries. It was in this region that he would spend the rest of his life.

The religious teaching of the Scottish Kirk emphasized man's sinfulness and depravity, but the young poet, influenced by the writings of Locke, Hume, and Pope, took a more optimistic view of the human state. He was handsome and, according to his contemporaries, fun loving and sociable. He enjoyed singing and dancing and wherever he lived he found his way regularly to taverns for convivial evenings with his many friends. In these settings, he joined in all the social activities but he could also be seen scribbling notes that presumably later found their way into poems. Burns once said "Freedom and whisky gang together" and he certainly drank his share, although one of his biographers wrote he was "never too drunk to write a letter" at the end of the evening. Indeed, in one of his poems he referred to "O thou, my Muse, guid auld Scotch Drink."

Any consideration of the life of Robert Burns cannot ignore what many consider his most evident personal trait—a pervasive interest in women. He found women, many of them, enormously appealing, and most of them in turn found him attractive. He was, in a word, a womanizer and his life story on one level is mainly one of a web of tangled relationships with women. It began shortly after the death of his stern, moralistic father, when he impregnated a local Mauchline girl. There would be many more. In fact, nine of his 14 children were born out of wedlock. To his credit, he always acknowledged these offspring, usually provided (within his meager resources) for them, and adopted several of them into his own home. His illegitimate children were born to local peasant girls in the various places he lived, but he also formed a few romantic liaisons with women whose social standing matched or even exceeded his own, in Edinburgh and elsewhere. Some of these latter relationships may not have been overtly sexual, but they led him to write unabashedly passionate poems and letters. One especially noteworthy relationship involved a young married woman he met in Edinburgh with whom he exchanged long letters brimming with passion over several years. When finally they parted for good, he composed a poignant, bittersweet poem, *Ae Fond Kiss*, regarded by many as one of the greatest love poems ever written:

> *Ae fond kiss, and then we sever,*
> *Ae farewell, and then forever!*
> *Deep in heart-wrung tears I'll pledge thee*
> *Warring sighs I'll wage thee.*
> *Who shall say that Fortune grieves him,*

When the star of hope she leaves him?
Me, nae cheerful twinkle lights me;
Dark despair around benights me.

The most remarkable, and certainly the longest, of his many affairs with women involved Jean Armour, a Mauchline lass from a good family. She fell in love with him and in a few months was pregnant. Her family was scandalized but, even though, he made clear he had no intention of marrying, she refused to place any blame on him. About that time, Burns departed for Edinburgh and Jean was left alone to deliver and care for twins, a boy she named Robert and a girl. A year or two later, he returned for a visit and she conceived again, bearing a second set of twins nine months later. Unhappily, both died shortly after birth and then the older girl died, so while Burns was basking in the glittering light of Edinburgh, Jean struggled alone with her remaining child, the young Robert. Their relationship rekindled when Burns moved to Dumfries and eventually they married and had several more children. So ultimately Jean won out—except that Robert, being Robert, continued his promiscuous ways. A barmaid at the local pub gave birth to his child, which Jean promptly took into her own home nine days before she herself gave birth. She commented nonchalantly, "Our Rabbie should have had two wives." Jean Armour was in some ways as remarkable a person as was Robert Burns and her benevolent acceptance of his behavior almost defies understanding.

One of Burns' early associates characterized him as "the only man I ever saw who was a greater fool than myself when woman is the presiding star." What role, if any, did this apparent addiction to sex play in the genius that was Robert Burns? Was it merely that these two independent characteristics happened by chance to occur in the same person? Or was there some sort of relationship between high sexual energy of this type and creative genius? There are many Burns devotees who believe the latter. Burns himself seemed to, for he wrote that he "never had the least thought or inclination of turning Poet until I got heartily in Love, and then Rhyme & Song were, in a manner, the spontaneous language of my heart." He expressed his feelings best in one of his most familiar lyrics:

O my luve's like a red, red rose,
That's newly sprung in June.
O my luve's like a melodie
That's sweetly play'd in tune.

As fair though art, my bonnie lass,
So deep in luve am I:

And I will luve them still, my dear
Till a' the seas gang dry.

Burns' choice of writing poetry in the Scots dialect is especially noteworthy, given that at the time it was considered uncouth. He certainly knew proper English—his letters were usually written in it—so the choice presumably reflected national pride. It sometimes makes his poems difficult to understand today, for the Scots dialect is not very familiar to the modern ear, but it gives his poetry a distinct lilt and resonance that add to it immensely. His collected works—poems, lyrics to traditional tunes, and letters—fill four volumes, a prodigious output by any standard but one that almost defies imagination when recalling that it was all written in about 20 years and all at times when most hours of the day were preempted by activities necessary for making a living.

Burns wrote of his native land in poems that stir the breast of every loyal Scot, as much today as two hundred years ago. One of his more famous pieces invoked the names of Scotland's greatest heroes, William Wallace and Robert the Bruce, in what has become the country's unofficial national anthem:

Scots, wha hae wi' Wallace bled,
Scots, wham Bruce has aften led,
Welcome to your gorie bed,
Or to victorie!

A child of the enlightenment, Burns was firmly committed ideals of liberty, freedom, and equality. The American and French revolutions occurred during his life and he found much to admire in both these cataclysmic events. Once, in a large gathering of establishment figures, when a toast to British Prime Minister William Pitt was proposed, Burns suggested raising glasses to "the health of a better man, George Washington." This was certainly a bold act for a governmental employee and expressing such radical sentiments got him into difficulties several times, forcing him to recant more than once. His ideas about egalitarianism and equality were also influenced by Freemasonry, an important part of his life, and found their famous expression in A Man's a Man:

A prince can mak a belted knight,
A marquis, duke, and a' that;
But an honest man's aboon his might'
Guid faith he mauna fa' that!.

15

But Robert Burns was much more than a nationalistic poet or even more than one who articulated the ideals of freedom and equality characterizing the Age of Enlightenment in the late 18th century. It was his genius to find ways of using the most ordinary and mundane of situations and objects to plumb the very depths of the human experience. What could be earthier than lice and mice? Yet Burns used these two vermin to express profound insights. In To a Louse (subtitled On seeing One on a Lady's Bonnet in Church) he made a fundamental observation about one's inability to be objective about oneself:

> O wad some Power that giftie gie us
> To see oursels as ithers see us!
> It wad frae mony a blunder free us,
> An' foolish notion!
> What airs in dress and gait wad lea'e us,
> An' ev'n devotion!

In To a Mouse (subtitled On Turning Her Up in Her Nest with the Plough, November 1785) he took the occasion to describe, in an oft-quoted phrase, the uncertainty surrounding even the most careful planning:

> The best-laid schemes o' mice and men
> Gang aft agley,
> And leave us nought but grief an' pain,
> For promised joy!

Illness and Death

Most of what is known about Robert Burns' health, as indeed most of the information concerning his life in general, comes from his astonishingly voluminous correspondence. Through nearly all of his adult life, he wrote a vast number of letters to many different people, and those that survive— some must have been lost or destroyed—constitute an important part of his literary legacy as well as major biographical sources. With respect to his health, as early as 1784 when he was only 25, he mentioned "fainting fits & other alarming symptoms of a Pleurisy or some other dangerous disorder which indeed still threaten me." Later, in the winter of 1789-90, he complained of fatigue and seems to have been depressed enough that he was unable to keep up his writing for a time. Yet until virtually the end he was able to continue the punishing physical labor that characterized his life, first as a hardscrabble farmer and later as an excise man.

By late 1794 and early 1795, the subject of his health came up more and more frequently in his letters. Unfortunately, he was not very specific in describing his symptoms, mentioning only "having been in poor health" or "being ill in bed for many weeks." He did use the term "rheumatism" several times, suggesting joint pain. Of course, 18th century medicine, especially in rural Scotland, was not very scientific and the only diagnosis he reported his doctors having given, "flying gout," is unhelpful. What is clear from his letters, however, is that his health was failing and by the early summer of 1796 the situation had become critical. In a June letter he referred to his "protracting, slow and consuming illness" and the next month he wrote of having been ill for eight to ten months, which would put the onset sometime around October 1795.

His doctor, William Maxwell, who was also a good friend and a neighbor, treated him with mercury injections and, when there was no improvement, suggested a therapy then fashionable in Scotland: drinking water from one of several wells thought to be therapeutic, accompanied by bathing in the sea. Thus, on July 3, 1796, Burns made the nine-mile journey to Brow Well on the coast where he took the waters and daily or more often immersed himself in the cold waters of the Solway Firth. On July 10, he wrote three noteworthy letters: one to his father-in-law asking that help be sent for his wife, Jean, who was expecting a baby in two weeks, another to his brother Gilbert saying "I am dangerously ill, & not likely to get better," and the third to a friend indicating he recognized that the end was near ("An illness which has long hung about me in all probability will speedily send me beyond that bourne whence no traveller returns.") To a friend he happened to see at this time, he asked, "Well, madam, have you any commands for the other world?"

On July 18 he returned to Dumfries in a borrowed carriage, unrestored and scarcely able to walk without assistance. A neighbor who saw him reported, "He had gone away very ill and returned worse." He took to his bed and gradually slipped into unresponsiveness, punctuated with episodes of delirium. Early in the morning of July 21, he died. The funeral, held four days later, had a military flavor because of Burns' membership in the local militia. Following a service of the Church of Scotland, two regiments escorted the cortege, accompanied by the Dead March from Saul; a rifle company fired a volley over the coffin; and the body of Scotland's greatest poet was buried in St. Michael's Kirkyard. Later in the day, Jean went into labor and delivered their ninth child, a boy named Maxwell after the doctor. Twenty-one years later, when Burns' genius had become widely appreciated, a public subscription raised money for an appropriate monument, the coffin was exhumed and relocated to an elaborate Grecian mausoleum elsewhere in the

17

kirkyard. The ever-faithful Jean, who survived her husband by 38 years, was also buried there, as were several of their children. Thus, in the end, Jean came to have her Rabbie all to herself, perhaps some measure of reward for her devotion and unimaginable forbearance.

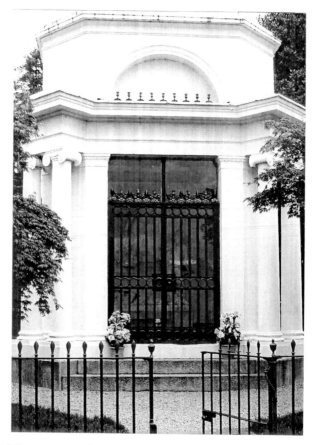

Figure 2.2 Burns mausoleum, St. Michael's Kirkyard, Dumfries, Scotland

At his death, Burns was famous throughout Scotland and, to a lesser extent, England, but little known outside the British Isles. However, within two or three decades of his death his fame had spread beyond Britain, eventually extending literally around the world. Burns clubs were established in almost every country and continue to this day, meeting regularly to read and discuss the poet's works. Each year on the date of his birth, January 25, Burns devotees around the world gather for an evening of Scottish food and libations and Burns poetry. No other writer, indeed no other historical figure, has his birthday remembered in this way.

The nature of Robert Burns' health and specifically the cause of his death, although much speculated upon, are not known with any certainty. Medicine of the late 18th century was still pretty much in its Dark Ages, almost totally lacking in any scientific basis. There were no accurate diagnostic aids such as the stethoscope and the concept of diseases based on structural or functional abnormalities was still 50 or 75 years away. Thus, diagnoses such that made by Dr. Maxwell, "flying gout," lack specificity or meaning.

In the wake of the poet's death, his followers recognized the need for a biography. The person chosen for this task, James Currie, seemed well qualified for the assignment, for he was a medical doctor and had a broad understanding and appreciation of Burns' literary genius. With all available Burns papers and letters available to him, he produced a four-volume biography that quickly became, and has remained, a standard source of Robert Burns' life and legacy. Currie's motives were pure (e.g., he gave all the profits of his biography to Jean and the children), but he had one enormous blind spot that consumed him—he was a vehement foe of alcohol and, like many moral zealots, he believed that anything sinful must necessarily be harmful as well. Thus, he concluded that Burns died of alcoholism, a judgment accepted uncritically by the next wave of biographers, but since largely discredited. Deaths related to excessive alcohol intake most commonly come from cirrhosis of the liver, and there is absolutely no evidence that Burns suffered from anything like this. Another important counter to any alcoholism theory is the simple fact that he could hardly have sustained his prolific literary output if impaired to any significant degree.

Certainly Burns drank, at times to excess, and his writings indicate occasionally that he worked to curtail the habit (e.g., while acknowledging that "occasional hard drinking is the devil to me," he observed that "against this I have again and again bent my resolution, and have greatly succeeded"). However, he also regarded alcohol as a source of his creativity, more than once referring to whisky as his "Muse," something that inspired his writings. Undoubtedly, Burns would agree with Winston Churchill who, when criticized about his drinking, responded: "I have taken more out of alcohol than alcohol has taken out of me."

Currie also suggested that "accidental disease," an 18th century euphemism for venereal disease, was involved in his death, but again no evidence whatsoever exists to support this contention. To be sure, Burns was promiscuous, even after he married, and so he was at risk for sexually transmitted diseases, but none of his writings give any suggestion that he was infected in this way. More importantly, syphilis being the only fatal venereal disease, his wife lived a long and healthy life and none of his surviving children manifest any evidence of congenital syphilis. Therefore, it seems clear that Currie's conclusion that Burns had a sexually transmitted disease was simply another reflection of the biographer's strident moralizing.

Another proposal, one coming mainly from romantic writers of the 19th century, but also retained by a few more recent biographers, is that the poet simply worked himself to death. To be sure, he was certainly no stranger to hard physical toil. He worked literally from dawn to dusk, trying to scratch a living from farming in several different locations, and in the end his efforts were defeated by poor soil, bad weather, and recurrent blights. When he attained his job as excise man, it gave him a steady income but it still involved long hours of brutally hard work, along with his continued agricultural activities. There is an old adage that "hard work never killed anyone," and it is true. Moreover, Burns was able to keep up with enormously demanding tasks and still find time at night for his voluminous writings. Farming caused him much anguish and depression, but there is no reason to think physical labor injured his health.

Sir James Chrichton-Browne in 1926 made the first serious and detailed analysis from a modern medical perspective, concluding that Burns died of chronic rheumatic heart disease and its complications. In rheumatic heart disease, one or more of the heart's four valves are damaged so that the flow of blood through the heart is impaired The basis of Chrichton-Browne's conclusion is not very clear but one of the important pieces of evidence seems to have been a description of the poet as a teenager, given by his brother Gilbert: "At this time he was almost constantly affected in the evenings with a dull headache which at a future period of his life was exchanged for a palpitation of the heart, and a threatening of fainting and suffocation in the night time." This picture is consistent with acute rheumatic fever, which could have led to chronic valvular rheumatic heart disease some years later.

Subsequent analyses by other physicians—Anderson in 1928, Vincent in 1954, Goodall in 1959, and Buchanan and Kean in 1982—all accepted the conclusion that Burns probably had rheumatic heart disease and it most likely caused his death. Nowhere in the description of Burns' terminal phase can specific symptoms or signs common with end-stage heart failure, such as difficulty breathing or erratic pulse, be found. However, what is recorded is quite consistent with the varied and ubiquitous course of a complication known as infective endocarditis in which bacteria attach to a damaged heart valve and then shower small particles of infected material into the blood stream. Therefore, the medical consensus seems to be that Burns died of chronic rheumatic heart disease with development of infective endocarditis on one or more damaged heart valves.

Medical Perspectives

Rheumatic fever is an immunologic disease arising from the body's reaction to infection with the streptococcus, a bacterium that commonly causes "strep throat." From one to five weeks after streptococcal infection, a small proportion of affected individuals become ill with fever, joint and muscle pains, and occasionally cardiac symptoms, consistent with a diagnosis of acute rheumatic fever. This condition can, in rare circumstances, be fatal, but usually it clears over the course of weeks or months. Then, years later, the individual with a past history of acute rheumatic fever may be found to have a heart murmur, indicating chronic damage to one of more of the heart's valves.

The heart has four main valves, one in each of its two outflow tracts and one in each of the two communications between the atria and ventricles. These values serve the general purpose of promoting blood flow in the desired direction when the valve is open and preventing back flow in the undesired direction when the valve is closed. Thus, when the atrium or ventricle contracts, the valve opens and the force of the contraction propels blood forward; after the contraction, the valve closes to prevent blood from leaking back. The net result of this intricate system is to keep blood flowing properly.

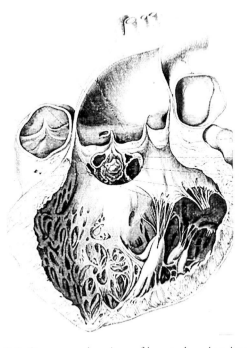

Figure 2.3 Cut-away drawing of heart showing its valves
(Courtesy of National Library of Medicine)

Valves may be damaged (and chronic rheumatic fever is the most common mechanism by which they are damaged) in two ways. They may become stenotic, meaning they do not open fully and the contraction-propelled blood flow is reduced in much the same way that a nozzle on a garden hose, if tightened down, results in less water coming out the end of the hose. The second type of valvular damage is one in which the valve does not close fully after the contraction, permitting some of the blood already expelled to leak back into the atrium or ventricle; this is called insufficiency. Both types of damage can exist in the same valve, a combined stenosis-insufficiency, and one or more valves may be damaged as a complication of rheumatic fever.

The atrium or ventricle pumping against a stenotic valve will have to work harder and harder to overcome or compensate for the defect and keep the rate of blood flow as normal as possible. The heart being composed almost entirely of muscle, the atrium or ventricle will then enlarge under the burden of this increased work, in much the same way a body builder in a gym builds up his or her body muscle with repeated weight lifting. In the case of the insufficient valve, the leakage of blood back into the atrium or ventricle with each contraction means there is an abnormally large volume, which causes the atrium or ventricle to dilate and also to work harder in an effort to move the high blood volume. In either case, after years of this excessive strain on the heart due to abnormal blood flow, eventually the heart become unable to meet the increasing demands, and its contractions begin to weaken. This end stage is known as heart failure. Other complications of rheumatic valvular heart disease include formation of blood clot(s) in a dilated heart chamber, usually an atrium. Parts or all of these clots can break off, enter the blood stream, and ultimately occlude a vessel to a vital organ elsewhere in the body.

A particularly serious complication of valvular heart disease is bacterial or infective endocarditis, the condition in which an area of bacterial infection forms on a valve. Bacteria occasionally gain access to the blood stream (e.g., fairly frequently with dental treatment or childbirth) but in the normal vascular system there is no place they can "catch on" to set up an infection, and the body defense mechanisms soon get rid of them. However, a damaged heart valve provides a site where circulating bacteria can attach and, once this has happened, the attachment can be extraordinarily hard to eradicate. An area called vegetation is formed and little pieces of it, which consist of infected material, break off and go throughout the body where they lodge in small blood vessels, occluding the vessels and setting up small abscesses. The treatment is a prolonged course of antibiotics administered intravenously (and therefore requiring hospitalization). This therapy is usually but not always curative; without treatment, the condition is nearly always fatal.

The last half-century has witnessed a marked decrease in the frequency of rheumatic fever and its complications. The principal reason for this is prevention of acute rheumatic fever by proper treatment of streptococcal infections. Giving penicillin (or, in those allergic to penicillin, another appropriate antibiotic) to individuals with streptococcal sore throat for ten days is highly effective in preventing rheumatic fever and its subsequent complications. There has probably also been some benefit from improvement in general health, nutrition, and living conditions, since rheumatic fever formerly was especially prevalent in crowded urban living situations. Thus, rheumatic heart disease, formerly a common type of cardiac disease, has become quite unusual, at least in medically advanced cultures.

For those who do have damaged heart valves, the incredible advances in cardiac surgery of the last 50 years have provided means of correcting the damage, sometimes by actually replacing the valve with a mechanical equivalent. Another improvement in outcome has resulted from the near-elimination of bacterial endocarditis by the practice of prophylactic antibiotic treatment of individuals with valvular heart disease when they are exposed to any manipulation with a chance of bacteria gaining bloodstream access, such as dental treatment or childbirth.

As a result of all of these factors, death from rheumatic heart disease has become a rarity. In 2004 (the latest year for which statistics are available), for example, only 3,248 deaths in the United States were attributed to rheumatic heart disease, representing only one-half of one per cent of deaths due to all types of heart diseases.

What if Robert Burns had been born 200 years later, in 1959? He probably would not have developed acute rheumatic fever because any streptococcal infections would have been treated with penicillin, and therefore he would not have had rheumatic heart disease. Even if he did develop the cardiac complication because of untreated streptococcal infection, he would eventually have had corrective surgery. Bacterial endocarditis would have been treated, and probably cured, with antibiotics. Thus, there can be reasonable confidence that had Burns lived in the modern era, he would have survived well beyond 37 years. His output of verses, songs, and letters would presumably have been much, much greater. But one cannot help but wonder—rhetorically—whether a healthy Burns would have been able to reach inside his soul and express such profound and fundamental insights of human existence?

<u>SOURCES</u>

McIntyre Ian. *Dirt and Deity:* A Life of Robert Burns. HarperCollins. London. 1995.

Bentman Raymond. *Robert Burns.* Twayne Publishers. Boston. 1987.

Grimble Ian. *Robert Burns.* Lomond Books. London 1994.

The Complete Poems and Songs of Robert Burns. Geddes & Grosset. New Lanark, Scotland. 2000.

Chrichton-Browne J. *Burns from a New Point of View.* Hodder and Straughton. London. 1926

Buchanan WW, Kean WF. Robert Burn's (sic) illness revisited. *Scot Med J* 1982;27:75-88.

www.american heart.org/presenter.jhtml?identifier+4712. Accessed May 5, 2008

CHAPTER 3

GEORGE GORDON, LORD BYRON AND MALARIA

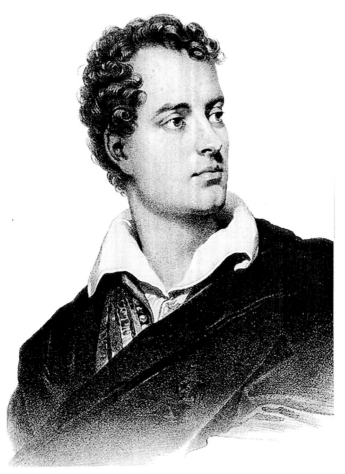

Figure 3.1 George Gordon, Lord Byron

"Mad, bad, and dangerous to know" was how one of his many paramours described the Sixth Lord Byron of Rochdale. It was an apt characterization, for Byron's behavioral aberrations far surpassed mere eccentricity, although they gave him, at least to some, certain engaging and even charismatic qualities. His sexual exploits, which involved men as well as women, scandalized early 19th century England and forced him into exile for the last decade or so of his life. Yet, in spite of these characteristics—maybe even because of them—he became arguably the most important of Romantic poets. Wealth and aristocracy, having come to him unexpectedly, freed him from the necessity of earning a living and supported an extravagant lifestyle of romantic adventuring, giving rise to a form of immortality conveyed in the term "Byronic hero." But there had to be more than affluence and interesting experiences to explain poetry that is as much respected and loved today as it was nearly two centuries ago. He died during his 37th year following a short illness, acquired while on a quixotic mission in support of Greek independence, believed to have been malaria. A parasitic disease, malaria has been virtually eliminated in developed countries by mosquito control measures, but on a worldwide basis it remains a major public health problem.

Biography

The future poet the world would know as Lord Byron was born in London on January 22, 1788. His father, Captain John Byron, nephew of the Fifth Baron Byron of Rochdale, had acquired his military rank along with the nickname "Mad Jack" while serving with the Coldstream Guards. The poet's mother, Mad Jack's second wife, was a Scottish aristocrat, Catherine Gordon of Gight. Both families represented ancient lineages, but many ancestors on both sides were known more for erratic habits and violent behavior than for any kind of noble actions. Mad Jack's main interests were gambling, women, and high living. His first wife, also an heiress, died shortly after giving birth to a daughter, but not before Jack had run through her wealth. Quickly remarrying, he proceeded to work on spending his new wife's money. Mad Jack was not present for the birth of his son, having gone to France to avoid creditors, and he appeared only intermittently thereafter, usually in attempts to wheedle money from his wife. He died in France, probably a suicide, when young George Gordon Byron was three years old.

The young widow and her son returned to her native Scotland, settling in Aberdeen. Her resources exhausted, they lived in rented quarters. The boy attended Aberdeen Grammar School, where the curriculum was almost entirely in Latin, and very early he demonstrated a consuming interest in reading. When he was six, there came a sudden and unexpected change in the family fortunes; the grandson of the current Fifth Lord Byron was killed in battle in Corsica and young George Gordon became heir to the barony. Four years later he succeeded his great-uncle as the Sixth Lord Byron, a title that brought the family estate, Newstead Abbey, and some 3200 acres of land in the vicinity of Nottingham. It seemed the family's financial problems were over, or at least should be. Mother and son moved to England, where they found Newstead Abbey in rather dilapidated condition due to inattention and exploitation by the recently departed Fifth Lord. In 1801, the young lord went to the famous school, Harrow, where his record was decidedly mixed. However, the move offered a welcome opportunity to develop an identity separate from his emotionally unstable mother.

Finishing Harrow in 1805, Byron matriculated at Trinity College, Cambridge where, although colleagues later could not recall him ever attending a lecture, he eventually was granted a degree. Over the two years of intermittent enrollment he drank heavily, lived riotously, and established friendships with a set of witty Cambridge men who fostered his preoccupations with classical literature and progressive politics. He also had two collections of poetry printed privately and, in 1807, published his first poetry volume, *Hours of Idleness*. Attaining his majority in 1809, he gained sole control of his inheritance and he took his seat in the House of Lords. However, his reception there was cool and he soon lost interest in trying to influence the political process, although his political interests would revive from time to time.

Also in 1809, Byron and a friend of Cambridge days embarked on an early 19th century version of the grand tour, with travel and extended stays in Portugal, Spain, Malta, Greece, Albania, and Turkey. It marked the beginning of an attraction to the Mediterranean world that would remain strong for the rest the poet's life. The trip also provided opportunities for excitement and adventure and included many diverse and exotic sexual experiences, both heterosexual and homosexual. Finally and perhaps most importantly, during these travels he began what many regard as his masterpiece, the long epic poem *Childe Harold's Pilgrimage*, the first two cantos of which he had completed when he returned to London after two years' absence. His homecoming was marred by several bereavements within a few weeks: his mother, a good friend from Harrow, and a young man who had been his homosexual lover at Cambridge. Sobered by these losses, he revised many portions of *Childe Harold's Pilgrimage*, deleting flippant and satirical passages and changing the overall tone to a meditative and even melancholic view of civilization in decline.

With publication of cantos I and II of *Childe Harold's Pilgrimage* in 1811, Byron, in his own words, "awoke one morning and found myself famous."

He quickly became one of the Britain's most popular and recognized persons, rivaling even the Duke of Wellington. His social activities at Newstead Abbey involved revelry on the grandest of scales. The toast of London society, he was much in demand for every kind of social function, for the world, in the words of one of his new friends, had gone "stark mad about Childe Harold and Byron." Despite such heavy social commitments, he maintained a high level of productivity, writing and publishing several lengthy poems during the interval of 1811-1815. In the House of Lord he aligned himself with the Whig opposition to the Tory government, giving speeches on liberal causes such as workers' rights in his home district of Nottinghamshire, Catholic emancipation in Ireland, and Parliamentary reform.

Byron seemed to be possessed of an extraordinarily high level of sexual energy. He clearly was bisexual. He had experienced homosexual relationships during his time at Cambridge, and perhaps even earlier while at Harrow, and an attraction to adolescent boys would reappear periodically. Byron was certainly aware of the very strict anti-sodomy laws in Britain at the time, prescribing severe penalties, even death, but there is no indication this risk represented much of a deterrent to him. At other times, he would be fervently heterosexual, and the period after his return from Europe was such a time. Byron's fame led to a series of romantic intrigues, most of them liaisons with aristocratic, often married women—beautiful, intelligent, talented, and daring women drawn irresistibly to the mercurial poet. But then he began an affair with Augusta Leigh that would lead to his fall from grace, or at least from public acclaim. It was not that Augusta was married—nearly all his paramours were—nor was there concern that the relationship was just another cursory and casual dalliance, for Byron would always say Augusta was his only true love. But Augusta was his half-sister, the product of his father's first marriage. English society might put up with homosexuality, promiscuity, and adultery, but incest was another matter. Augusta had a baby, her third, on April 15, 1814, and there has always been a question as to whether the father was her husband or her half-brother.

Byron's problems were compounded by persistent and pervasive financial difficulties. The income from his holdings was substantial, but not adequate to meet his extravagant lifestyle, and creditors hounded him constantly. His poetry, especially *Childe Harold's Pilgrimage*, was hugely successful commercially but it brought him no financial gain. Regarding literary earnings as beneath the dignity of a nobleman, he gave all his copyrights, at least in the early years, to a friend.

For all these reasons, by 1813 the bloom on the rose of Lord Byron's popularity had begun to fade. In what may well have been in an effort to address this image problem, the poet decided to marry. He proposed to Annabella Milbanke, a young and rather naïve woman with wealthy parents, who first rejected his proposal and then agreed when he persisted. The wedding took place in early January 1815 and the match was in trouble from the beginning. The new Lady Byron had doubts about her husband's morals and loose attitudes toward religion—he had previously characterized her as having an "awkward kind of correctness"—but she thought she could reform him. The first few months involved some degree of mutual affection but soon Byron became intent on shocking his bride, often at times when he had been drinking heavily, by recounting his many and varied sexual activities. Eleven months after the marriage, Annabella gave birth to a daughter who was named Augusta Ada; the first name was presumably intended to remind everyone of the new father's most notorious love affair and the child would always be called Ada. A month later, Lady Byron had had enough and she and the child moved in with her parents. Her husband, after a few half-hearted attempts at reconciliation, agreed to permanent separation, sending his wife a poem that was part lament, part accusation:

> *Though my many faults deface me,*
> *Could no other arm be found,*
> *Than the one which once embraced me,*
> *To inflict a cureless wound?*

The scandal of the separation added to persistent rumors of "unnatural practices" made England an uncomfortable place for the poet who had been lionized just a couple of years earlier. His indebtedness compounded his problems, and so in April 1816 he chose exile across the English Channel, never to see his native land again. He sought refuge in work, beginning on canto III of *Childe Harold*. One of his early verses expresses his creative urge and quest to find in poetry the intensity he needed to fuel his life:

> *'Tis to create, and in creating live*
> *A being more intense, that we endow*
> *With form our fancy, gaining as we give*
> *The life we image, even as I do now.*
> *What am I? Nothing; but not so art thou,*
> *Soul of my thought!*

Along with a retinue of servants and hangers-on, Byron toured France and Germany, eventually settling in a villa on the shores of Lake Geneva, adjacent to another villa occupied by Percy Bysshe Shelley and his wife Mary. Shelley and Byron shared many characteristics—both were poets, idealists, radical political thinkers, and skeptics about religion—and their relationship, one of mutual admiration, would be important to each over the next several years. Accompanying the Shelleys was Mary's stepsister, Claire Clairmont, whom Byron had impregnated in a brief affair in London a few months previously. It was certainly an odd consortium and one that many back in England viewed as scandalous, but over the summer of 1816 it produced several works destined to become enduring classics of English romanticism: Mary Shelley's *Frankenstein*, Percy Shelley's *Mont Blanc* and *Hymn to Intellectual Beauty*, and Byron's canto III of *Childe Harold* and *The Prisoner of Chilon*.

Continuing his European wanderings, Byron settled in Venice, a place whose sophisticated and hedonistic atmosphere suited him. He continued his amorous activities, first with the beautiful young wife of a merchant and then a succession of mistresses, some noble, some bourgeois, and some low-born, that he claimed numbered "at least two hundred." His attempts to emulate Don Giovanni ended in 1819 when he met and fell in love with Teresa Guiccioli, the innocent bride of a 58-year-old count. It was a relationship that would prove to be the most sustained and satisfying of Byron's life. Count Guiccioli tolerated the situation at first, but eventually some solution was needed and Teresa's father arranged a separation sanctioned by the Vatican. Leaving the carnival atmosphere of Venice, Byron and Teresa settled in Ravenna. Byron presumably remained faithful to Teresa from here on, except for a homosexual affair while he was separated from her near the end of his life.

The period 1819-1822, when Byron's attachment to Italy strengthened as his bonds to his native England weakened, was one of intense creativity and enormous productivity for the poet. Having completed *Childe Harold* canto IV, he began work on what would be his other masterpiece, *Don Juan*, using the technique of ottava rima he had recently discovered. This poetic technique, used by early Italian poets, follows the pattern abababcc and most considered it too difficult for English because of that language's fewer rhyme-words. But Byron was able to master it. Other aspects of his life also began to improve. For the first time, he attained financial stability; the sale of Newstead Abbey and substantial income from his publications (at some point he began keeping this money) provided a steady income that was adequate to support a lifestyle as extravagant as his. However, tragedy struck in 1822. Allegra, his five-year-old illegitimate daughter by Claire Clairmont, died of typhus at her convent school and Shelley drowned while boating in a lake. Byron moved to Genoa where he provided some assistance to the widowed Mary Shelley and from where, in July 1823, he sailed away on what would be his last adventure.

Byron's literary output was enormous by any standard. His *Complete Poetical Works* comprises seven volumes and an edited and indexed version of his complete letters and journals runs to no fewer than twelve volumes. He was also an extraordinarily versatile poet, responsible for an array of works classified as lyric, satire, tale, and drama. With such an output as this over about 20 years, one might assume that poetry flowed easily from his pen; John Ruskin, an English poet of the next generation, said, "Byron wrote, as easily as a hawk flies." But this is a vast over-simplification, for he was actually very disciplined in his writing and existing copies of his original manuscripts demonstrate repeated reworking and editing as he searched out just the right words. Of his many works, the two that stand out as his masterpieces are *Childe Harold's Pilgrimage* and *Don Juan* and it is on these that his literary legacy must be assessed. Both are long narrative poems: part travelogue, part philosophical treatise, and part commentary on contemporary affairs. The first is considered largely autobiographical, emphasizing the poet's melancholic, alienated feelings, whereas the second uses a fictional lothario in a seemingly lighter, gayer, and wittier setting.

How is Byron to be judged? He was certainly famous during his lifetime, and that reputation has hardly dimmed since. His influence on concepts of creativity has been acknowledged by many luminaries extending across the full range of the arts—writers, artists, and composers, both his contemporaries and those coming years after him. He is the only poet to rate a separate chapter in Bertrand Russell's *History of Western Philosophy*. Around him and his life would develop the cult of the "Byronic hero," a noble yet flawed man of action and adventure, with little regard for convention or propriety, but with a certain redeeming virtue—in contemporary terms, a James Dean-type of rebel without a cause. Yet his behavior, in particular his sexual morality, anathematized him to many in his own time, a judgment that has certainly not softened. Controversial as he is, Byron was certainly one of the greats—and many would argue the greatest—of the remarkable group known as Romantic poets.

Illness and Death

Given Byron's intensely romantic character, it seems almost inevitable that he would meet his end in some idealistic quest. The most idealistic quest available at the time was the Greek struggle for independence from the Ottoman Turks. It wasn't ideal—the Greeks had more than their share of unreliable or incompetent leaders, petty infighting and rivalries, and widespread venality—but the pull of classical Greece was enough for Byron. He had, after all, written of Greece in canto III of *Don Juan*:

The mountains look on Marathon,
And Marathon looks on the sea;
And, musing there an hour alone,
I dreamed that Greece might still be free.

It was enough to lead Byron to outfit, largely at his own expense, a ship and company that sailed from Genoa in July 1823. The expedition stopped for a time at Cephalonia, an island under a British Protectorate, and then proceeded to Missolonghi, a marshy town on the mainland. During these months, Byron was entirely in male company, and his homoeroticism was rekindled by his 15-year-old Greek page, who returned his advances reluctantly if at all. At Missolonghi, where the party arrived in early January 1824, he was greeted as a hero, but he soon discovered many obstacles to his goal of capturing a nearby Turkish fortress, and an attack he hoped to lead never materialized. Moreover, the site was unpleasant and unhealthy, surrounded by stagnant lagoons and pelted by heavy winter rains. While waiting, Byron wrote letters and a few poems, rode, shot, and tried to keep his troops from fighting over rank and precedence. Within a few weeks, his health began to deteriorate. In February he suffered an epileptic-type of convulsive seizure, but he seemed to recover fully and most authorities regard it as unrelated to his subsequent illness.

On April 9, after a long ride in the rain, Byron came down with a fever, attributed initially to a common cold. His two doctors, one Italian and the other Dutch but educated in Britain, were both quite inexperienced and one was a bit of a charlatan as well. They urged bleeding, at the time a fashionable treatment for illnesses with fever. The patient refused, asking "Have you no other remedy than bleeding? There are many more die of the lancet than the lance." Over several days, his condition steadily worsened, although he felt well enough to go for a long ride on one occasion. He weakened and complained of headache and joint pains, as well as chills and fever. Ultimately, he gave in to his doctors' repeated importunities and consented to be bled. Leeches were applied to his temples and substantial quantities of blood (said to have been "a pound" on each of two occasions) were withdrawn However, the treatment did not produce any improvement and the set of medical consultants, now augmented with two well known local doctors, now tried other therapies—purgatives, opium, ether, and blisters applied to the body. As the poet's condition deteriorated, the sickroom scene became a chaotic mess, with no one in charge and agitated directions and orders shouted in various languages, none of then intelligible to anyone except perhaps the shouter.

By April 18, Easter Sunday in the Greek Orthodox calendar, it was clear to all that Byron was dying. He was intermittently delirious and even when he seemed rational he spoke, sometimes in English and sometimes in Italian, a jumbled litany of instructions, laments, and prophecies. A consistent theme, according to one observer, was his agony for Greece: "Poor Greece . . . I have given her my time, my money, and my health; what could I do more? Now I give her my life." That evening, he said "I must sleep now" and lapsed into a coma. Twenty-four hours later, at 6:15 PM on April 19, the poet was dead.

Byron's physicians performed an autopsy the next day but, probably because of their inexperience, it was not particularly revealing: the membranes covering the brain were thickened, the heart seemed large, and the liver appeared small and cirrhotic, but none of these gave any hint as to the cause of death. The postmortem dissection conflicted with Byron's expressed wishes, and in another way his desires were apparently ignored: his body was embalmed and prepared for shipment back to England, denying him the soldier's grave he had envisioned in one of his last poems, written on his 36th birthday:

> *Seek out—less often sought than found—*
> *A soldier's grave, for thee the best;*
> *Then look around, and choose thy ground*
> *And take thy rest.*

Byron's death drew attention to the Greek cause and inspired a new wave of support among western cultures. To the Greeks he became a national hero, every bit as much as if he had died in battle, and a funeral service in Missolonghi on April 22 was follow by a prolonged period of public mourning over the whole of Greece. To this day, the English poet is commemorated throughout the nation by road- and place names, statues, and paintings. The question of where his body should come to rest elicited as much controversy as the poet himself had in life, but ultimately the decision was to return it to England. After embalming, the body was placed in a casket through which numerous holes were drilled, then the coffin was put in a larger container containing 180 gallons of alcoholic spirits, and the whole thing was shipped by boat to a harbor where a ship waited to sail for England on May 25. On numerous occasions in ports and other land sites along the way, there were salutes involving discharges of cannon and musketry.

As the ship carrying Byron's corpse made its way to England, the poet's supporters envisioned a triumphant public burial in Westminster Abbey. However, there was considerable opposition by those who could neither forget nor forgive Byron's scandalous living. Ultimately, the Dean of Westminster ruled out an Abbey burial. The ship reached the Thames estuary on June 29 and several days later docked in London, to be met by a delegation of friends, admirers, and dignitaries. The funeral cortege drew crowds as it made its way north from London to its destination at Hucknall Torkard, a few miles from Nottingham, where the poet was buried in the Byron family vault under the parish church. There were subsequent campaigns for a memorial in Westminster Abbey, but none succeeded until 1969, nearly a century and a half after his death, when Parliament decided that, whatever his sins in life, his poetry merited him a plaque in Poet's Corner.

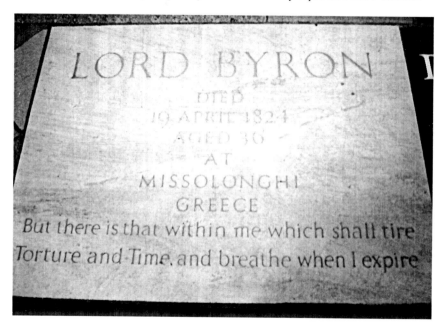

Figure 3.2 Byron plaque in Westminster Abbey
(Courtesy of Dariush Afshar)

What illness overtook Byron in the spring of 1824 and what specifically caused his death? It was an acute condition, probably lasting only a week or ten days from onset to fatal termination, and accompanied by fever, characteristics suggesting strongly some sort of infectious disease. Immediately after his death, the physicians involved attempted to place blame on the patient himself for refusing their recommended bleeding for so long. In addition to being incredibly self-serving, this judgment is about as wrong as any could be. Bleeding may have been common and even standard treatment in the early 19th century, but it was totally ineffective and, especially when the amount withdrawn was large, detrimental to health by itself. In Byron's case, the amount of blood withdrawn, by leeches or by directly cutting a vein was considerable, estimated recently at 2.5 liters, corresponding to nearly half his total blood volume, over some 60 hours. Bloodletting was certainly a major contributory cause of his death, by weakening his ability to fight infection, and might even have been responsible primarily.

Early biographers of Byron suggested typhoid fever as the cause of his death, but there is little evidence to support this diagnosis. Indeed, the specific statement in the autopsy report that the stomach, liver, and kidneys were healthy argues strongly against it. What is considered the most authoritative examination of the question came in 1924, on the centenary of the poet's death, when two eminent British physicians, one a Nobel laureate, examined the available records independently. They each concluded, one perhaps more assuredly than the other, that the most likely diagnosis was an unusually virulent form of acute malaria, a disease transmitted by mosquitoes. A recent medical re-analysis concurred in this finding. Unfortunately, the autopsy made no mention at all of the condition of the spleen and, if malaria were involved, the spleen would almost certainly have been enlarged. However, the place where Byron lived from early January to mid-April 1824 is a low-lying marshy area on the Gulf of Patras, adjacent to a lagoon and at the time utterly lacking in sanitary facilities. This area of southern Greece, one of the experts noted, is characterized by malaria cases beginning in early spring, as mosquitoes infected from the previous autumn come out of hibernation. Another recent medical appraisal suggested Mediterranean tick fever (an infection spread by dog ticks) as perhaps more likely than malaria. Nevertheless, the accepted diagnosis continues to be malaria.

Byron's medical history includes two other conditions that, while not involved in his death, are essential to any understanding of the man. One of these was lameness due to a foot and ankle deformity, causing him to walk with a peculiar sliding gait. The exact nature of the problem is not known with certainty, but it was undoubtedly congenital. Some have suggested it represented a mild form of cerebral palsy but more likely it was the common club foot deformity in which the foot is turned down and inward so that the affected individual walks on the ball and outside of the foot. Byron's mother took him as a child to see a number of practitioners, most of them quacks, about this problem and the boy was subjected to various treatments that were both painful and ineffective. Later, he had a special boot made and he wore it nearly all the time. Curiously, there is some confusion among the various observers as to which foot was involved, but the best evidence is that it was the right.

Byron was very sensitive about his deformity, once commenting about the difficulties in overcoming "the corroding bitterness that deformity engenders in the mind, and which sours one to all the world." Not surprisingly, he went to great lengths to conceal it, presumably to protect the heroic, virile image he wanted to project. An avid horseman throughout his life, he regularly boxed and fenced and he had played cricket for Harrow. His favorite sport was swimming, one little impaired by his deformity, and he took special pride in having swum the Hellespont, a distance of four miles of cold water and strong currents, on his first European trip in 1810. Friends, associates, and servants learned quickly to avoid any mention of his deformity. Even on his deathbed, when he acquiesced in his doctors' wishes for blister therapy involving applying glass globes to his legs, one to each leg, he asked that they apply both to his left leg, presumably to avoid exposing his deformity.

The other and even more interesting of Byron's medical conditions involves his mental and emotional status. Everyone with whom he came in contact described him as a person of tumultuous and contrasting passions who could variously be idle and furiously productive, ascetic and libertine, aristocratic and republican, idealistic and crass, tempestuous and pensive. This picture of wild swings from the highest of spirits to the lowest melancholy is classic for the mental illness known presently as bipolar disorder, formerly termed manic-depressive psychosis. An important feature of bipolar disorder is its familial nature, and here again Byron meets the criterion. In fact, he quite likely inherited a double dose of whatever causes the disease, for both maternal and paternal lineages are littered with individuals whose behavior was nothing if not bizarre. His father, as noted earlier, was known as "Mad Jack" and he ran through the fortunes of two wives, before (probably) committing suicide. Byron's great uncle was known as the "Wicked Lord" and, but for his title and wealth, his behavior would have probably have landed him in prison or an insane asylum. The inheritance from the maternal side was, if anything, more dangerously unstable. The poet's mother was given to violent moods and unpredictable behavior and he once referred to her in a letters as "a compound of derangement and folly." Her ancestry, going back to early Scottish history, included many individuals who died violently, from either suicide or execution for murder.

Some authorities suspect a specific linkage between bipolar disorder and artistic creativity, and bipolar disorder is unique among psychiatric illnesses in this regard. Careful examination reveals that many of history's greatest poets, authors, playwrights, painters, and composers exhibited behavior (including suicide) and/or had family histories of bipolar disorder or one of its milder variants. The association seems especially common in the case of poets and there are few well-known poets who did not have at least some suggestion of bipolar disorder. Perhaps this is because, while all creativity is enhanced by elevated and expansive mood and ability to focus effort over long periods, in poetry there is a special need for fluency, the ability to rapidly conceive words and test them in constructing expressions and sentences. Byron, regarded as the classic example of the poet with bipolar disorder, seemed well aware of his condition. He made many references to madness in his poems and he once wrote in a letter "We of the craft are all crazy. Some are affected by gaiety, others by melancholy, but all are more or less touched."

Medical Perspectives

The disease we call malaria has afflicted man from the beginnings of history and perhaps earlier. Signs of it have been found in Egyptian mummies and the disease was described quite clearly in ancient Greek writings. It is believed to have caused the death of Alexander the Great in Mesopotamia in 323 BC. The name comes from the Italian mal'aria meaning "bad air" and Romans thought it came from swampy fumes. As a cause of illness and death, it may not have been dramatic like such cataclysms as bubonic plague or Spanish influenza, but its steady and unrelenting presence led one eminent authority to say that is "has caused the greatest harm to the greatest numbers."

Malaria is caused by infection with a parasitic organism, microscopic in size but somewhat larger than bacteria, of the genus *Plasmodium*. Four species of *Plasmodium* can infect humans, but the *falciparum* species causes the most severe disease. It is responsible for almost half of human cases and 95% of deaths. The vector for all *Plasmodium* transmission is the female Anopheles mosquito, which acquires the organism by consuming blood from an infected individual and then transmits it by biting an uninfected person. In its new host, infective forms of the parasite are carried by blood to the liver where, reproducing rapidly within liver cells, they cause the cells to rupture. Returning to the blood, new infective forms attack red blood cells and multiply wildly, circulating with the blood and often causing the red cells to rupture and spill their contents. If the newly infected individual is bitten by a female Anopheles mosquito, these infective forms will isolate in the mosquito's salivary glands where they can infect the next person the mosquito bites.

Signs of the disease typically begin at the end of the liver phase of the cycle, some ten days to two weeks after the primary infection. Fever is the most common symptom and the classic picture is that of cyclic paroxysms, with a shaking chill lasting an hour or two, then high fever for some hours or a day or two, and ending with drenching perspiration and the temperature falling to normal or even below. However, this classic history of recurrent chills and fever, with the individual feeling quite well between episodes, is not always observed and, when not present, the diagnosis can be difficult. Other symptoms include tiredness, weakness, aching joints and muscles, nausea, and diarrhea. In its severest form, falciparum malaria involves the brain, so impaired consciousness or other neurologic symptoms are especially ominous. The acute symptoms, especially chills and spiking fever, seem to coincide with rapid destruction of red blood cells and this process can sometimes be so extensive as to cause kidney failure due to release of free hemoglobin from the destroyed blood cells. The diagnosis is made by microscopic examination of a blood smear showing characteristic Plasmodium forms.

The organism causing malaria was identified in 1880 and a few years later it was demonstrated in the stomach of a particular mosquito species. Thus, by the end of the 19th century, the role of mosquito transmission was appreciated, and this knowledge led to concerted efforts at malaria control through eradicating mosquito breeding grounds, first during the building of the Panama Canal and later elsewhere throughout the world. In temperate climes, mosquito control measures proved effective and the disease virtually disappeared, although it persisted in tropical and sub-tropical regions.

Along with control by draining mosquito-breeding areas, public health measures such as insect repellants, screens, and netting proved quite effective in controlling malaria in developed countries, especially those in non-tropical areas. In the 1920s, the United States Public Health Service, with financial support from the Rockefeller Foundation, launched an aggressive mosquito control program, first in Arkansas and then in other southern states. The results were astonishing; within three years malaria was virtually eliminated from the United States. Today, in the U.S. and similar countries such as those in Northern Europe, cases are encountered very rarely and then nearly always after having been acquired during travel to tropical areas.

The success of mosquito control programs improved markedly with the development and widespread usage of the insecticide DDT, which proved enormously effective and by the 1960s had raised the prospect of wiping out malaria. However, overuse of this effective agent effectively dashed these hopes, first by the development of DDT-resistance and then by the recognition that the insecticide, while not toxic to humans, can cause adverse environmental effects. Rachel Carson's *Silent Spring*, published in 1962, painted an alarming picture of reproductive damage to peregrine falcons, sea lions, and salmon that led to DDT being outlawed for agricultural use in many countries. Although exceptions were made for malaria control in highly endemic areas, DDT had acquired a bad name, and the dream of eradicating the disease became forlorn. Finally, chronic under-funding of other mosqui-to control measures added to the problem and as a result there have been recent increases in malaria frequency. Thus, on a worldwide basis, malaria remains a major public health problem in more than a hundred countries, mostly in sub-Saharan Africa, Central and South America, the Middle East, and Asia, regions accounting for over 40% of the earth's population. The World Health Organization estimates that each year there are about 300 million new cases and more a million malaria-related deaths. Children under age 5 seem especially susceptible to the disease and account for the majority of deaths. Presumably, older children and adults have sufficient immunity from earlier attacks that they can usually hold new infections in check.

Malaria is unusual, perhaps even unique, among diseases in that an effective form of therapy was known long before there was any understanding of the nature of the illness itself. In the early 17th century, Spanish colonists in Peru and Ecuador found the indigenous peoples of South America treating fevers by having affected people chew on the bark of the cinchona tree, which they called "quina quina." The results were dramatic and Jesuit missionaries brought this "miracle drug" back to Europe, where malaria was quite prevalent, in about 1632. The active component of cinchona bark was isolated during the early 19th century and given the name quinine. Thus, quinine has been the mainstay of both prevention and treatment for nearly four centuries. It is still used today in severe cases of *falciparum* malaria. However, quinine is short acting and carries considerable risk of complications, particularly involving hearing and the heart, so in all but the most severe cases it has been replaced with newer and safer drugs.

Atebrin, developed in the 1930s as a successor to quinine, was widely used for both prevention and treatment during the Second World War, especially in the Pacific theater. Atebrin is not used today because, while tolerated better than quinine, it still has undesirable side effects. Chloroquine, the next agent synthesized, came into usage toward the end of World War II and initially proved highly effective and well tolerated. Unfortunately, the organism developed resistance to the drug; in some areas as much as half of *P. falciparum* became resistant to chloroquine. A number of other drugs have been developed in recent decades, but most seem plagued by drug resistance. Combination of two or more agents seems at present the best approach to dealing with this problem. There is considerable current interest in a Chinese herbal preparation, artemisia, that seems promising and is currently under intense testing as part of a combination drug therapy. Nevertheless, because of drug resistance plus weakening mosquito control programs, malaria seems to be on the rise and authorities recently designated it the most serious public health threat worldwide.

Turning now to the other aspect of Lord Byron's medical history, bipolar disorder, the question of an association with creativity remains especially controversial. Are bipolar disorder and creativity linked, perhaps by common genetic characteristics? Are individuals with tendencies to emotional extremes likely to choose artistic careers? Is bipolar disorder an asset to creativity? The answers to these questions are not known. At present, the most authoritative word on the subject comes from Professor Kay Redfield Jamison of Johns Hopkins University: "Most people who suffer from manic-depressive and depressive illnesses are not unusually creative and they reap few benefits from their experiences of mania and depression; even those who are highly creative usually seek relief from their suffering. Nevertheless, some affected persons believe a linkage between their disorder and creativity exists."

There have been major advances in understanding and treatment of bipolar disorder and related conditions over the past 50 years. To be sure, there is no cure, but careful, appropriate drug treatment has permitted many afflicted with the condition to lead relatively normal lives. Drugs for bipolar disorder fall into two categories, mood stabilizers and antidepressants, the former intended to prevent or treat mania and the latter for depression. The mainstay of drug therapy is lithium, a mood stabilizer introduced in 1949 and proved in many subsequent studies to improve the course and outcome of the illness. Some anticonvulsant drugs, especially valproate and carbamazine, have proved to be useful alternatives in patients unable to tolerate lithium or unresponsive to it. Used singly, lithium seems to be more effective than valproate in preventing suicide. Various antidepressants are available for treating the depressive phase. It is essential to monitor pharmacological therapy—what drugs are given and in what doses—very closely, for a characteristic of bipolar disorder is for those afflicted with it to slip from manic to depressive phase and vice versa in very subtle ways.

As noted earlier, at least some poets, writers, composers, and artists afflicted with bipolar disorder report that drug treatment of their psychiatric disorder, particularly with lithium, inhibits their creativity. Those who feel they do their best work while in mildly manic phases describe lithium as acting as a brake on their ability to express themselves and taking away their creative drive. However, scientific studies of the issue have yielded mixed results; while some have found some lowering of cognitive functions (decreased ability to learn, concentrate, and memorize), others have found that the drug seems to increase creativity as often as decreasing it. Though the scientific community is uncertain about the relationship between drug treatment and artistic-creative expression, many affected individuals seem convinced of an adverse influence and some even discontinue taking prescribed drugs, at least during periods of intense productivity.

If it should turn out that treatment of the disorder in the process limits creativity, an ethical dilemma exists with respect to when and whether they should be prescribed and how strongly patients should be urged to take them. Potentially, there is an even more serious ethical issue in the offing. Given its strong familial predisposition, it seems likely that bipolar disorder is genetic in origin and there could be some linkage between it and creative genius. If the affected gene(s) can be identified, prenatal diagnosis and genetic engineering will almost certainly follow. In such a scenario, the world might get rid of a debilitating psychiatric disorder, one that causes much pain and anguish and many cases of suicide, but if a linkage with creativity exists, the medical advances could also foreclose the possibility of another Byron, or another Poe, Eliot, Pasternak, Conrad, Faulkner, Hemingway, Schumann, Gauguin, van Gogh, or any of a number of the world's creative geniuses.

What then would have been the outcome if Lord Byron lived today, rather than nearly two centuries ago? Assuming the diagnosis of malaria was made, there is every reason to believe that proper drug therapy, started early and almost certainly involving a combination of agents, would be effective. His clinical picture was that of severe disease, requiring parenteral therapy with quinidine gluconate and either clindamycin or a tetracycline. He may have actually received cinchona bark because it had been available in Europe since the early 17th century and was often given where there was any kind of fever. But if he did get it, it was certainly too little and too late. With respect to his psychiatric condition, he would be given lithium and probably other drugs as well and these would like have controlled his wide mood swings. However, they might also have limited his phenomenal poetic productivity.

SOURCES

MacCarthy Fiona. *Byron: Life and Legend*. Farrar, Straus and Giroux. New York, 2002

Garrrett Martin. *George Gordon, Lord Byron*. The British Library Writers' Lives. Oxford, New York, 2000

Graham Peter W. *Lord Byron*. Twayne Publishers, New York, 1998

Jamison Kay Redfield. *Touched with Fire: Manic-depressive Illness and the Artistic Temperament*. Simon and Schuster, New York, 1993

Dale Phillip Marshall. *Medical Biographies: The Ailments of Thirty-three Famous Persons*. University of Oklahoma Press. Norman. 1952

Editorial: The centenary of Byron's death. BMJ 1924;1:724-6

Mills AR. The last illness of Lord Byron. *Proc R Coll Phys Edinb* 1998;28:73-80

Scarlett EP. Lord Byron: "The pilgrim of eternity." *Arch Intern Med* 1963;112:616-20

Baird JK. Effectiveness of antimalarial drugs. *New Engl J Med* 2005;32:1565-77

Schou M. Artistic productivity and lithium prophylaxis in manic-depressive illness. *Br J Psychiatry* 1979;135:97-103

www.who.int. Accessed June 14, 2007

CHAPTER 4

THE PRINCESS CHARLOTTE OF WALES
AND DEATH IN CHILDBIRTH

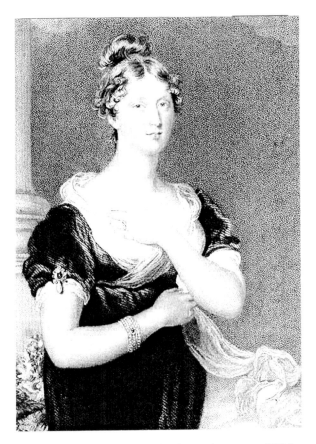

Figure 4.1 The Princess Charlotte Augusta of Wales

The marriage and subsequent pregnancy of Charlotte Augusta, Princess of Wales, led to great rejoicing in early 19th century Great Britain because, as George III's only legitimate grandchild, Charlotte represented the future of the monarchy. But joy turned to anguish when, following a very long and difficult labor, the Princess was delivered of a stillborn infant, and then a few hours later she died herself. This double tragedy, which set in motion a series of events that would profoundly influence the course of world history, illustrates how dangerous childbearing has been throughout most of human existence. Until about 70 years ago, the risk of a woman dying in childbirth, even in developed countries such as the United States, was nearly one in a hundred. After peaking about 1930, the risk began to fall and, once the decline started, the rate of fall was phenomenal, so that by 1980 it reached one in 10,000 live births. The increasing safety of childbirth is unquestionably the 20th century's most remarkable development as far as health is concerned, at least in developed countries. In less developed societies, where health care is lacking, the risk remains appallingly high.

Biography

Princess Charlotte's story actually begins with her grandfather who became King of Great Britain and Ireland as George III in 1760. His reign was a long one, lasting officially until his death in 1820. He experienced episodic mental breakdowns, portrayed in the popular play and movie *The Madness of King George,* and in the last few years his illness became severe enough that a Regent was appointed to rule in his place. Nevertheless, for more than 40 years, George III was one of the world's dominant figures, playing key roles in such important historical events as the American Revolution (e.g., his name appears prominently, and not very favorably, in the Declaration of Independence), the French revolution, and the Napoleonic wars.

George III had seven sons and five daughters. The eldest, the Prince of Wales (later Prince Regent and still later George IV) rebelled against his father's strict rules and lead a wild and dissolute life. A womanizer who ate, drank, and gambled to excess, he secretly married a commoner; however, the marriage was illegal because the Marriage Act stipulated that, as an heir to the throne, he required the King's permission to marry. Ultimately, he agreed to let his father and the government choose a bride, probably because the agreement provided coverage of the enormous debts he had accumulated in his playboy activities. The bride selected was Caroline of Brunswick, an obscure German princess, and she and her groom never met until their wedding day in April 1795. The marriage was a disaster from the outset. The Prince, raised in the world's most cultured aristocracy, was appalled with what he saw as a boisterous, crude, and ill-mannered woman from a minor German court. Following an elaborate wedding, bride and groom spent the night together and, legend has it, never shared the same bed thereafter In any case, it is a fact that Caroline gave birth 9 months to the day after the wedding, on January 7, 1796. It was a girl and she was baptized Charlotte Augusta by the Archbishop of Canterbury a month later. The Prince and Caroline spent the rest of their lives in a continuous acrimonious dispute.

The Princess Charlotte grew up under the most difficult of circumstances. Her parents were consumed with their constant battling and each strove to use the child against the other. It reached such a state in 1804 that the King finally stepped in, proposing that Charlotte live with him so he could supervise her upbringing and oversee her education. The Prince of Wales agreed as long as his wife would have no say in the child's life, a condition that was unacceptable to the King, as well as, of course, to the girl's mother. Negotiations proceeded over several months, with the entire Royal Family involved on one side or the other, until finally an agreement was hammered out. Charlotte would remain under her father's care, living next to him when he was in London, but when he was away (which actually was most of the time) she would reside at Windsor Castle under the King's supervision. Her mother would have visitation rights but these would be very limited in both frequency and length. The King would nominate her governess but the Prince retained final right of approval.

With the constant tug-of-war involving Charlotte, it is easy to understand how she grew up more than a little neurotic. Talkative, high-spirited, and given to emotional outbursts, she constantly sought the affection denied her by her parents. She was tall and, if not exactly a stunning beauty, had a certain handsome, regal appearance. One of the young soldiers attached to the court wrote that "her eyes were blue and very expressive and her hair was abundant and of that peculiar light brown that merges into the golden." As she grew into adulthood, she developed definite democratic leanings, making her very popular with the people. This popularity contrasted with that of her father whose political leanings were much more conservative and, with his dissipated life and corpulent appearance, the Prince was anything but admired. It is said that when they went for carriage rides, Charlotte was cheered but the Prince met with stony silence. There was, of course, another reason the British people found her attractive: she represented the assurance of succession of the monarchy. Moreover, she was the only hope, for although George III had many children and some of them had children, Charlotte was his only grandchild born of a legal marriage.

As the Princess approached adulthood, the matter of her marriage assumed increasing importance. By this time, King George's mind had gone entirely and his eldest son had become Prince Regent, meaning that Charlotte, as the heir apparent, became Princess of Wales. Her father, always more interested in controlling her than in loving her, proposed Prince William of Orange, the son of King William of The Netherlands, as an appropriate suitor. His choice was motivated entirely by political considerations, the cementing of an Anglo-Dutch alliance. Charlotte acquiesced initially, but later broke the engagement when she learned that the marriage contract required her to live six months each year in Holland.

A few months later, some European diplomats met in London to celebrate the victory over Napoleon. One of them was the 26-year-old, handsome Prince Leopold of Saxe-Coberg, a younger son of a minor German prince, and he mounted a campaign to attract the attention of the Princess of Wales. It took a while—there were other candidates for her hand and he needed to ingratiate himself with members of the Royal Family and the ministers of state—but ultimately his quest was successful. The Princess Charlotte of Wales and Prince Leopold were married in a glittering ceremony at the Prince Regent's residence on May 2, 1816.

The marriage turned out to be as successful as that between Charlotte's parents had failed. It was, indeed, a union made in Heaven, in contrast with one made in Hell. Charlotte and Leopold had sharply contrasting personalities: she was voluble, emotional, and tempestuous while he was mature, urbane, and cultured—exactly what was needed to tame an impulsive, wild princess who had always sought affection but never found it until marriage. To be sure, their contrasting personalities led sometimes to friction but Leopold, experienced as a diplomat and schooled in the continental tradition, knew exactly how to deal with his bride. Their spats always ended in the same way: with flaming cheeks and sparkling eyes, Charlotte would say, "If you wish it, I will do it." Leopold would invariably reply, "I want nothing for myself; when I press something on you, it is from a conviction that it is for your interest and for your good." Leopold also worked successfully to improve her manners, which were atrocious for a member of royalty, and to develop her self-control.

The couple divided their time between Camelford House in London, a wedding present from Parliament, and a country home in Surrey. Seen often at cultural affairs and church services, they became tremendously popular with the London crowds. The affection of the people for their handsome Princess and her Prince Consort reflected in large part the couple's model demeanor, especially as it contrasted with the antics of many other Royal Family members, which the public found embarrassing and even disgusting. Percy Bysshe Shelley, in his poem *England in 1819*, minced no words in describing the public's general view of the Royals: "Princes, the dregs of their dull race, who flow through public scorn, mud from a muddy spring."

Charlotte had two miscarriages in the months following her marriage, but in 1817 there was a third pregnancy and it seemed to be proceeding well. An official announcement, after the danger of miscarriage had passed, let to universal rejoicing. Not only was the public elated for the popular couple, but there was the simple fact that the child Charlotte carried would be third in line for the throne and would guarantee the succession for another generation. This preoccupation with royal succession might seem odd to a country lacking a monarchial tradition, such as the United States, but it has been characteristic of kingdoms, especially Britain and, before Britain, England. The people shared this preoccupation, less perhaps because of concern for the present royal line but more in the knowledge that disputed succession had often led to imposition of a foreign monarch or, worse yet, civil war. For the Royal Couple, the rest of the Royal Family, and the people of the British Empire, it was a time of happy anticipation.

The doctor given the task of leading the medical team caring for this vitally important pregnancy was Sir Richard Croft. He had been closely associated with Thomas Denman, one of London's best known and most influential obstetricians, having married Denman's daughter and having practiced with him. Denman was the leading advocate of ultraconservatism in obstetric management, articulated mainly in his text *An Introduction to the Practice of Midwifery*, which went through many editions since first published in 1788. Denman promulgated a number of restrictive rules, including one that forbade the use of forceps to deliver the infant except as a last resort, after all else had failed. In the last edition of his text, published in 1816, Denman made very clear his disdain for obstetrical forceps: "It would have been happier for the world if no instrument of any kind had ever been contrived for, or recommended in, the practice of midwifery." Forceps represented the only means available at the time to hasten birth, labor-stimulating drugs not having been developed and cesarean section not really feasible because it virtually always led to death of the mother.

Sir Richard's practice included the highest level of society and he had attended several women of the aristocracy in their labors. Thus, at least on paper he appeared ideally suited to his important assignment. Privately, however, some of his colleagues wondered if his prominence did not come more from his family connections than his knowledge and ability, and a few regarded him as timid and lacking in self-confidence.

Princess Charlotte's pregnancy progressed reasonably well. She complained at times of headache but there were no alarming symptoms. Sir Richard prescribed a rather restricted diet, but he did suggest walking for exercise. Bleeding was a common form of treatment in those days and the Princess was bled on at least three occasions. She went beyond term, causing the public to become anxious, but reports issued from the palace indicated that she continued to be well. Finally, at 7 PM on Monday, November 3, two weeks and a day past the calculated due date, the bag of waters ruptured and labor began.

<u>Death and the Aftermath</u>

Princess Charlotte's labor was long and progress excruciatingly slow. Finally, an examination at 9 PM on November 4 indicated that the head had moved deep in the pelvis and the cervix (or opening of the uterus) had dilated completely. Complete dilatation marks the end the first stage of labor, which in this case lasted 26 hours, compared with the usual 10-12 hours. It was now the second stage of labor (i.e., from complete cervical dilation through delivery of the infant) and the rate of progress was, if anything, slower. By evening of the 5th, 48 hours from the onset of labor and 24 hours since the second stage began, the head could finally be seen on the pelvic floor and at 9 pm the infant was born. A 9-pound male, the baby showed no signs of life and did not respond to efforts to "reanimate" him. The second stage of labor had lasted 26 hours, much longer than the usual 1-2 hours.

The placenta or afterbirth normally separates within a few minutes of the birth of the child. In Princess Charlotte's case, however, it did not separate completely and partial detachment led to excessive uterine bleeding over the next half hour. Sir Richard, after consulting with colleagues, decided to remove the placenta manually. This procedure involves inserting a hand and arm into the uterus and detaching the placenta from the uterine lining by insinuating the hand between the two. There was some difficulty, but eventually he was able to remove the placenta from the uterus, leaving it in the vagina in accordance with Denman's conservative teaching. There was more bleeding and the Princess complained of severe pain, so about 25 minutes later Sir Richard removed the placenta entirely. This was followed by a gush of blood.

The Princess at this point was reasonably comfortable and appeared as well as could be expected for a woman who had just completed a labor of some 50 hours, delivered a stillborn infant, and experienced some blood loss. She took some liquids orally. About midnight her condition seemed to change. She complained of nausea and then vomited and said she reported hearing singing noises in her head. Given a sedative because of restlessness, she slept for a half-hour or so, then awakened and seemed to be having difficulty breathing and thrashed about in her bed. Her pulse was reportedly weak but the rate remained below 100 beats per minute. Various medications were given, but at 2:30 in the morning of November 6, the Princess of Wales died.

Embalming was customary when a member of the Royal Family died and the embalming process involved removal of the internal organs, so it amounted to a reasonably complete autopsy. Done by the Sergeant Surgeons to the King the day after death, the postmortem examination's findings were a small amount of fluid around the heart, stomach contents of a quart or so of liquid, and the uterus distended with an estimated pound of clotted blood—not especially noteworthy in elucidating the cause of death. The infant was noted to be normal in every respect. The Princess and her son were buried together in St George's Chapel at Windsor Castle.

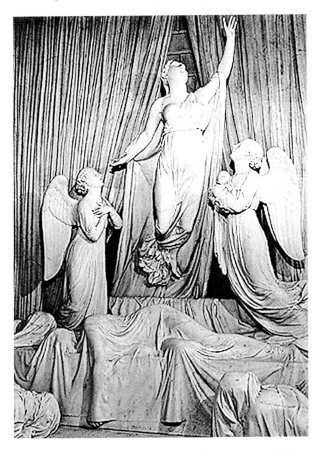

Figure 4.2 Memorial to Princess Charlotte and her infant son,
St. George's Chapel, Windsor Castle

The death of the unborn child was a tragedy, but Charlotte's death was a national catastrophe. It struck Britain and its Empire like a thunderbolt and the people's grief was as genuine as it was universal. Such an outpouring of public mourning had not been seen before and would not be seen again until the death of another Princess of Wales, Diana, 180 years later. The public expression of grief was followed quickly by anger and a search for those at fault for this national disaster. The official reports in the first few days were scanty and gave little information, leading to all sorts of wild rumors and charges of ignorance, mismanagement, and neglect on the part of the doctors. The allegations appeared in letters, often unsigned, in newspapers and they called for a public inquiry. Three weeks after the death, a detailed report in a leading London medical journal quieted the concern, at least to some extent.

The brunt of the criticism fell on the hapless Sir Richard Croft, even though Prince Leopold and The Prince Regent each issued statements that held Sir Richard blameless. Actually, his care was quite consistent with accepted management of the time. In retrospect, it is easy to see that delivery by forceps any time during the very long second stage of labor would likely have saved the baby and probably the mother, too. However, Sir Richard's hands-off approach was in keeping with the ultraconservative philosophy held by many, though admittedly not all, obstetricians of that day. Further, he had sought consultation with another member of the team who concurred with not using forceps. Sir Richard may have been indecisive and unsure of himself, but he was not guilty of a crime. He was characterized aptly by Louis Hellman, a well-known American obstetrician who analyzed the case in 1972, as "a lonely man in the delivery room upon whom the eyes of the world were focused, he had neither the fortitude nor the imagination to defy established tenets." Nevertheless, Croft took the blame and, depressed and despondent, he killed himself three months later, making the entire affair a triple obstetric tragedy.

The all-important question of succession now became an obsession. George III now had no legitimate grandchildren, so unless some came along, the line would die out with his children. Age, marital status, and the Marriage act (a law regulating royal marriages and succession) did not make prospects very encouraging. Of course, the Prince Regent, 59 and as overbearing as he was overweight, was already married and had been engaged in a violent dispute for all of the 23 years of his marriage to Caroline of Brunswick. Even if their relationship could be rehabilitated—an extremely unlikely happening—she was past the childbearing ago. His brothers, the Royal Dukes, were in childless marriages (two), long-term relations with mistresses (two), or marriages that conflicted with the Marriage Act (one); the youngest brother, 43, was still single. The five daughters offered even less promise; two were married but childless, two were secretly married against the provisions of the Marriage Act, and one was unmarried at age 49.

The two Dukes with mistresses quickly ridded themselves of their paramours and, along with the youngest, unmarried Duke, sought brides. With varying degrees of difficulty, appropriate candidates for all three were found in obscure German principalities. The eldest of the three, the Duke of Clarence married a young German princess in 1818 and the following year she gave birth to a premature infant who died a few hours after birth. A second pregnancy followed, also resulting in a premature infant who died at 7 months. The Duchess of Clarence had no more children. The next eldest, Edward, Duke of Kent, was aided in his search by Prince Leopold, the bereft widower, who suggested his sister Princess Viktoria. A widow with two healthy teenage children, Viktoria offered the powerful appeal of having proved her reproductive capacity. The match was made and pregnancy quickly followed, with the resultant birth of a female in 1819.

The monarchy was safe, at least for the time being, but things were not exactly smooth. Edward had always fought with his older brother, now Prince Regent and soon to become George IV, and the christening of the infant Princess when she was one month old almost degenerated into a brawl. The Prince Regent refused to let the baby be named Georgeana or Augusta, two prevailing royal names of the Hanoverian dynasty, and when the name Charlotte, his own deceased daughter, was proposed, he flew into a rage. Finally, there was agreement that she be called Alexandrina, after the czar of Russia. However, as she grew up and it became increasingly clear that she would someday be Queen, the name Alexandrina sounded too foreign. So she took one of her other names, that of her mother, with the spelling Anglicized. Thus, when she ascended to the throne of Great Britain and Ireland in 1837, it was as Queen Victoria.

Victoria's reign lasted 63 years, the longest ever of any British monarch, and it was by any standard a glorious one. The British Empire extended literally around the world, validating the claim that the sun never set on it, and Great Britain became the world's most powerful and influential nation. Queen Victoria was an integral part of this phenomenon, and in a real sense provided its driving force. British government was, by the 19th century, firmly a constitutional monarchy and the sovereign's power had clear limitations, but Victoria's influence went far beyond mere political authority. By her example and the sheer force of her will, she imposed a code of conduct and morality on the Royal Family, restoring the prestige of the Crown and establishing it as a symbol of public service and imperial unity. She gave her name to an age and to an ethical code that lasted long after her. The adjective "Victorian" may have somewhat of a pejorative connotation today, but Queen Victoria's positive influences cannot be doubted.

Through Victoria's six children and their marriages, her influence persisted long after her death in 1901. Her direct descendents played major roles in three of the four principals involved in World War I, a hundred years after Princess Charlotte's death: Victoria's grandsons occupied the thrones of Britain and Germany as George V and Kaiser Wilhelm, respectively, and Czar Nicholas of Russia was first cousin to both, as well as the husband of Victoria's granddaughter. World War II being a direct consequence of World War I, a case could be made that these two cataclysms of the 20th century occurred, at least when and how they did, as a consequence of the death of Princess Charlotte and her unborn son a century earlier. What would the course of world history have been if either or both of the two had survived? This is one of those questions that are as tantalizing as they are unanswerable.

Medical Perspectives

A stroll through any old graveyard will reveal a large number of tombstones of women who died in their twenties and thirties, many of them probably due to complications of pregnancy and childbirth. It is hard to put any kind of precise numbers on this risk because the tabulation of vital statistics (e.g., birth and death numbers and rates) did not really begin until the last century or so. But there is enough indirect evidence to substantiate that, for almost all of human existence, having a baby has been very risky business. Even as recently as 1900, childbirth ranked second only to tuberculosis in causing reproductive-aged women to die.

Maternal mortality is defined as death of a woman during or shortly after a pregnancy in which complication(s) of pregnancy or birth caused the death or at least played an important role in it. Conventionally, maternal mortality has always been expressed as the ratio between the number of deaths and the number of live births. The denominator for this statistic is live births, rather than number of total births or pregnancies, because live births are more likely to be recorded whereas stillbirths and pregnancies often go unreported. Originally, the maternal mortality rate was defined as the number of deaths per 1000 live births; as maternal deaths became less common, the base was changed, first to 10,000 and more recently to 100,000, in order to make the numerical rate easier to understand. For the sake of uniformity, this discussion will use the base of 100,000 live births.

Vital statistics were not kept on a nationwide basis in the early 19th century so there is no good way of telling how common deaths such as that of Princess Charlotte were. Some fragmentary information can be gleaned from statistics of individual hospitals (although the relationship of such figures to the general population is uncertain because the vast majority of childbirth confinements took place at home). The City of London Lying-in Hospital reported a maternal mortality rate (i.e., number of maternal deaths per 100,000 live births) of 990 for 1790 and 790 for 1810. Dublin's Rotunda, the world's first maternity hospital, reported a rate of 1150 for the eight-year period from 1807 through 1814 (for the same period, 4 % of infants were stillborn and 3 % of those born alive died within the first week of life).

In 1837, the Royal College of Physicians (London) and the Royal College of Surgeons (England) asked all medical professionals to supply certificates of death for all who died under their purview, such certificates to include the apparent cause of death. This marked the beginning of the collection of vital statistics. In the first year, 1837, the maternal mortality rate was 606 and it remained at approximately this level for a century. The situation was very similar in Scotland, where the records were probably even more reliable; from 1856 until about 1930, the maternal mortality rate fluctuated between 500 and 700. No reliable data from the United States exist before 1900, but for the first 30 years of the 20th century, the overall maternal mortality rate in the U. S. ranged between 650 and 850. Thus, a reasonable summary would be that, up until the end of the first third of the 20th century in the United Kingdom and the United States, two countries with rather good medical care for the time, somewhere between 600 and 800 women died for every 100,000 babies born alive. Put dramatically (though less accurately), up until about 70 years ago, a woman who conceived took a chance of about one in 125 to one in 165 of dying.

Sometime around 1930, things began to change and, once begun, the decline in maternal mortality was nothing short of phenomenal. The overall maternal mortality rate in the United States fell from 650 in 1930 to 380 in 1940, to 83 in 1950, to 37 in 1960, to 22 in 1970 and then to less than 10 in 1980. It has fluctuated around 8 and 9 over the past 25 years. Thus, in the relatively short space of 50 years, from 1930 to 1980 in the United States (and probably also in similarly developed Western nations), a woman's risk of dying in pregnancy and childbirth went from about one in 150 to one in 10,000. This represents a drop of around 99%, illustrated in the graph below, and no other index of public health has come close to this remarkable statistic.

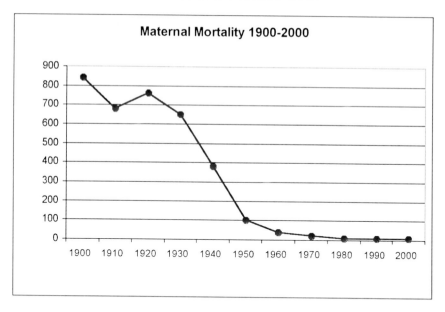

It is important to understand that this phenomenal increase in the safety of childbearing has been largely limited to developed nations. In the developing world, maternal mortality remains high, in many places appallingly so. According to a recent study by the (U. S.) Centers for Disease Control and Prevention and UNICEF jointly, the maternal mortality rate in 2002 in Afghanistan was about 1,600 and Afghani women face a cumulative lifetime risk of dying in childbirth of one in six.

What accounts for this astonishing increase in the safety of childbearing in developed societies over the relatively short space of half a century? Unquestionably, the major factor was the education of professionals involved in maternity care, based on enhanced knowledge and understanding of normal pregnancy and delivery and the abnormal variants along with a shift from home to hospital as place of birth. The concept of prenatal care—women being checked regularly throughout pregnancy—only began to gain acceptance in the early years of the 20th century. Improvements in other aspects of women's health undoubtedly played a major role. Specifically, availability and usage of family planning freed women from the tyranny of unrestrained reproduction, permitting them to bear children when they wanted and to avoid the increased risk that comes with too many pregnancies too often. Those whose medical condition made conception especially dangerous had the option of choosing to avoid the risk entirely. The availability of legal, safe pregnancy terminations virtually eliminated criminal abortions and their high rate of complications.

There was probably some effect of the improvement in general health and nutritional status that came with 20th century advances and certain specific developments such as antibiotics to fight infections and blood transfusions to treat hemorrhage, both developments of the 1940s, played important roles.

The major cause of maternal death in childbirth has always been the same, regardless of whether the frequency is high or low: excessive bleeding or hemorrhage, sometimes because of a complication in early pregnancy but usually during the first few hours after birth. To see how the problem of postpartum hemorrhage occurs and how it can be prevented and treated, it is necessary to understand something of the physiology of pregnancy and delivery. The placenta represents the sole means of supplying oxygen and nutrients to the fetus, as well as the only way of eliminating waste products. To carry out its functions, the placenta receives a large supply of blood from the mother, as much as a pint every minute in late pregnancy. This volume of blood comes through vessels that connect the maternal circulation to the placenta, vessels that enlarge progressively to provide the increased blood flow essential as pregnancy advances.

After the infant is born, the uterus, as a muscular organ, continues to contract, but because of the now-smaller size of the empty uterine cavity, its contractions effectively shear the placenta loose from its attachments to the uterine lining. Thus, usually within a few minutes of the infant's birth, the placenta separates from the inner surface of the uterus and is expelled through the cervix, into the vagina, and ultimately outside the body. Meanwhile, the site where it was formerly attached to the uterus has a number of large blood vessels that, until just a few seconds or minutes ago, carried large amounts of maternal blood to and from the placenta. Were there no way of controlling blood flow from these now-open vessels, every woman would bleed to death shortly after giving birth. Fortunately—and necessarily for the survival of the species—there is a way: the muscle fibers of the thick uterine wall are arranged in an interlacing manner so that when they contract they effectively squeeze the blood vessels shut, limiting blood loss normally to an average of about a pint or so.

Normal conditions do not always prevail, and sometimes blood loss can be much heavier than the customary pint. This complication of postpartum hemorrhage occurs in perhaps a tenth or so of births, most often when the uterine contractions after delivery are relatively weak and do not completely shut off the open blood vessels to the former site of the placenta. The uterus may not contract efficiently if it is "tired" because it has been contracting throughout a long labor, in much the same way a marathon runner is exhausted after completing the race. Abnormal bleeding after delivery can also occur when the uterus was previously over-distended during pregnancy (as with a very large baby or a multiple pregnancy), causing the muscle fibers to be stretched beyond the optimal length for efficient contraction postpartum. With modern methods of obstetric management, the threat of postpartum hemorrhage is lessened by giving a drug to stimulate the uterus to contract immediately after the infant's birth and, if necessary, repeating the treatment. Other and more powerful uterine stimulants can be given in cases that fail to respond. If blood loss continues at a high rate, blood transfusions can be given in replacement. In the very rare cases in which hemorrhage persists in spite of these measures, a surgical operation to tie off certain blood vessels or even remove the uterus can be done as a life-saving measure.

Traditionally, the second-leading cause of maternal death has been infection and, while death or serious complication due to infection has been reduced markedly by the availability of antibiotic drugs, the problem has not disappeared. Many different kinds of bacteria are present normally in the vagina. By contrast, there are normally no bacteria in the uterus, at least during pregnancy, so apparently the cervix represents an effective barrier. However, after a few hours of labor, especially if the amniotic membrane or bag of waters has ruptured, vaginal bacteria ascend into the uterus. There is normally no fever or other sign of infection, and delivery, when it occurs, treats the condition by providing drainage of any infected material. However, when labor goes on too long, the normal defense mechanisms can be overwhelmed, allowing frank infection to develop. This is an ominous event for both mother and baby. Infection invading the uterine wall can interfere with normal ability of the muscle to contract, prolonging labor even further. Further, the baby normally inhales amniotic fluid and with bacteria being inhaled, pneumonia may develop. Modern treatment with antibiotics can help prevent this sequence from beginning, and can certainly arrest it if it has occurred, but the most effective therapy for both mother and infant is for delivery to take place within a reasonable time of infection becoming apparent.

With this brief background, we can now return to Princess Charlotte and construct an analysis of what went wrong and why she and her unborn child died. The Princess may well have been anemic, and her resistance could have been lowered in other ways, by the restricted diet and repeated bleedings during her pregnancy. When she finally began labor, some two weeks after term, her uterine contractions were not very strong and this led to slowing of the course of labor. Somewhere in the middle of her 26-hour first stage, infection probably began in the uterus and this compounded the problem of inefficient contractions, leading to a long first stage and a very long second stage of labor. When the baby died is uncertain, but it was probably near the middle of the incredibly long second stage, due to pneumonia resulting from inhaling infected amniotic fluid.

Over the past 50 years, several obstetrical authorities have examined the case of Princess Charlotte. The most common conclusion has been that postpartum hemorrhage caused her death. There is much to support this explanation, particularly the long labor, but some of the details (e.g., the pulse rate consistently below 100 beats per minute) are not fully consistent with it and, moreover, it requires another condition to account for the infant death. Infection was at least an important secondary factor and could well have been primary; further, infection offers a reasonable explanation of the infant's death. Pulmonary embolus (a condition in which a blood clot goes from pelvic or leg veins, through the heart to occlude a major artery to the lung) has also been proposed. The Princess's terminal course, with difficulty breathing and restlessness, strongly suggests pulmonary embolus, but this condition leaves unexplained the infant's death and its association with prolonged labor is probably coincidental.

What would have happened if Princess Charlotte's pregnancy occurred today, rather than in 1817? Her prenatal care would have been different in that she would have been advised to eat a nutritious diet and supplemental iron would have been provided. Spontaneous labor would have been awaited, although perhaps some thought might be given to inducing labor as pregnancy continued past her due date. After labor did start, by 10 or 12 hours after the onset when it became obvious that progress was inadequate, and she would have been given small doses of intravenous oxytocin, a hormone-like drug that stimulates uterine contractions. In all likelihood, this treatment would improve the contraction pattern and hasten the end of the first stage. There would be concern if the second stage lasted for an hour or two, and a careful assessment would be made to determine the feasibility of an instrumental delivery. If conditions seemed proper for an easy delivery using forceps or vacuum extractor, that would be done. If the level or position of the baby's head made an easy forceps unlikely, or if earlier in the first stage progress arrested in spite of oxytocin, cesarean delivery would have been chosen. Either forceps or cesarean, as appropriate, would be done to effect immediate delivery if there were any evidence of fetal jeopardy (e.g., abnormal fetal heart rate patterns). If the woman evidenced any sign of infection (e.g., fever) or if a cesarean was to be done, antibiotic therapy would be initiated. After delivery, potent uterine-stimulating drugs would be administered, blood for transfusion would be kept readily available and the woman would be monitored carefully for hemorrhage.

If Princess Charlotte had received the kind of care standard today in a medically sophisticated country, one can say with virtual certainty that she and her infant son would be alive. But then, of course, the last 200 years of world history would have been vastly different.

SOURCES

Loudon I. *Death in Childbirth: An International Study of Maternal Care and Maternal Mortality 1800-1950.* Oxford University Press, Oxford, 1992

Holland E. The Princess Charlotte of Wales: a triple obstetric tragedy. *J Obstet Gynaecol Br Emp* 1951;58:905-19

Friedman AJ, Kohorn EI, Nuland SB. Did Princess Charlotte die of pulmonary embolus? *Br J Obstet Gynaecol* 1988:95:683-8

Achievements in public health, 1900-1999: Healthier mothers and babies. www.cdc.mmwr.gov/preview/mmwrhtml/mm4838a2htm. Accessed August 18, 2007.

Pearse WH. And, having writ, moves on: Presidential address. *Am J Obstet Gynecol* 1983;146:233-6.

CHAPTER 5

CHARLOTTE BRONTË
AND EXCESSIVE VOMITING OF PREGNANCY

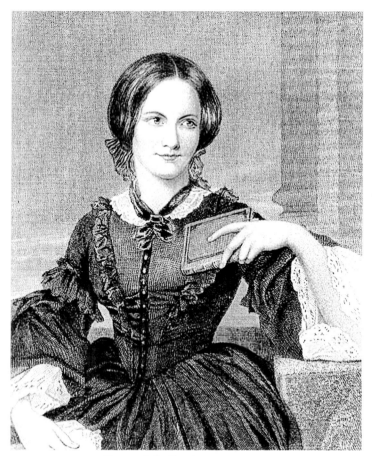

Figure 5.1 Charlotte Brontë

The literary world will never see another family like the children of an Anglican clergyman who lived on the windswept Yorkshire moors. The Brontës were also a family marked for tragedy, for the wife-mother and all six children died at early ages. Charlotte, the third child, was small and plain and had a drab personality. Moreover, she spent almost all her life in an environment that was anything but cosmopolitan and she was subservient to a demanding father. Yet she wrote prolifically—four romantic novels, many poems and short stories, and innumerable letters—and at least one of her novels, *Jane Eyre*, became a towering classic of English literature. Not until the age of 38, after watching each of her five siblings die of tuberculosis, did she marry; shortly thereafter she was seized with a protracted illness consisting mainly of vomiting, and she wasted away and died within two or three months. While the exact nature of her illness is not known, it most likely was excessive vomiting of pregnancy, an exaggeration of the "morning sickness" normally accompanying early gestation. The severe condition is still seen today but, treated with intravenous fluids and electrolytes along with drugs to suppress vomiting, it is never fatal nowadays.

Biography

Patrick Brontë, the eldest of 11 children of an illiterate farm laborer in Northern Ireland, very early in life caught the eye of a minister who sponsored the promising young man to go to Cambridge University to study theology and classics. Young Brontë prospered in the intellectual climate of Cambridge, where he became part of a movement committed to reforming the Church of England along more socially responsible lines. Ordained in 1806 when he was 29, he served several Yorkshire parishes as curate or assistant to the rector. While at one of them, he met Maria Branwell and, after a fairly brief courtship, they were married on December 29, 1812. Children came regularly: Maria in 1813, Elizabeth in 1815, Charlotte in 1816, Branwell in 1817, Emily in 1818, and Anne in 1820. Mrs. Brontë never really recovered from the last confinement and she was in poor health when Patrick received appointment as rector of the Church of Saint Michael and All Angels in Haworth. Elizabeth Branwell came from Cornwall to nurse her ailing sister, and she would remain after Maria's death in September 1821.

Haworth, new home of the soon-to-be motherless Brontë children, was on the edge of the Yorkshire moors. The winters seemed interminable, with pervasive dampness, howling winds, and frequent blanketings of snow. The residents of the parsonage at the top of the hillside town found themselves isolated socially as well as physically, for the population consisted of mill workers and The Reverend Mr. Brontë did not regard such people as suitable companions for his children. Brontë once wrote to a friend that he found himself "a stranger in a strange land" and the description applies to his children as well. The six children spent all their time together—reading, drawing, and writing—in the process laying the foundations of phenomenal creativity. Of course, Aunt Elizabeth Branwell was present and would remain part of the household until her death many years later, but she was more of a housekeeper than a surrogate mother. The father, while aloof, stern, and demanding, was highly intelligent and broadly knowledgeable in science, literature, art, and music, and he held daily instructional classes for his children. He was especially concerned for his five daughters, feeling that a sound education was essential to prepare them for what seemed to be best of their limited career options, that of a governess.

In 1824 the Cowan Bridge School for Clergymen's Daughters, about 45 miles from Haworth, opened. It seemed perfect and, moreover, the fees were modest, so The Reverend Mr. Brontë enrolled his four older daughters. But it proved disastrous. The conditions were abysmal: unheated, poor and inadequate food, harsh discipline and constant emphasis on sin and its inevitable punishment. Within a few months, Maria, the eldest, became ill with consumption (the 19th century term for tuberculosis), returned home, and died. Shortly afterwards, Elizabeth, the next, followed precisely the same course. The loss of two daughters within a year awakened their father to the true nature of the Cowan Bridge School and he brought Charlotte and Emily back to the family home at Haworth. Charlotte, now the eldest at age nine, mourned the deaths of her sisters and a profound sense of loss would haunt her the rest of her life.

For the four surviving Brontë children, education was now provided at home and, while unconventional, it was unbelievably rich, reflecting the father's commitment to a broad education and their own corporate creativity. They all read voraciously: newspapers, magazines, popular books such as *Pilgrim's Progress* and *Aesop's Fables*, classic texts from their father's library, and of course the Bible. They created elaborate imaginary worlds, wrote and acted plays, composed poetry, and drew pictures. Charlotte was especially close to her brother, a year younger, and the two stimulated each other and critiqued one another's efforts. Branwell clearly was favored by a father who regarded his only son as destined for greatness. To be sure, Branwell was intelligent, witty, and charming, but unfortunately his considerable natural talents were not matched by self-discipline.

After five years of this remarkable home environment, 14-year-old Charlotte needed to resume formal schooling to equip her for a career as a teacher or governess. In January 1831, she enrolled at the Roe Head School, a choice that proved much better than the earlier tragic experience. There were but ten pupils and two of them, Ellen Nussey and Mary Taylor, became Charlotte's life-long friends and correspondents. In fact, most of what is known today about Charlotte Brontë comes from the hundreds of letters she wrote to Ellen Nussey. Roe Head was ideally suited to Charlotte's insatiable thirst for learning. She delved deeply into history and geography, polished her considerable artistic abilities, and learned French and music.

After about 18 months at Roe Head, Charlotte returned to the Haworth parsonage to teach her sisters and brother. She also wrote poetry and turned out many landscape scenes and portraits (in pencil, ink, or water-color, but never in more expensive oil). In 1835, Charlotte took a teaching position and later became governess to two different households successively, but she found none of these positions satisfying. Eventually, she conceived the notion of her and her sisters, by now entering adulthood, starting a school in the Haworth parsonage. Such a venture would require more education and Charlotte was very interested in a European experience. Aunt Elizabeth Branwell agreed to finance a study-trip to Brussels for Charlotte and Emily and, in early 1842, the two girls left the north of England for the first time, spending a few days seeing the sights of London on the way to Brussels. Their father accompanied them and stayed long enough to get them settled at the Pensionnat Heger, a boarding school run by Monsieur and Madame Heger. The curriculum emphasized French, history, arithmetic, geography, and writing, "as well as all the skill in needlework which a well-brought-up young lady requires." Charlotte, and to a lesser extent Emily, reveled in the Continental culture and experiences. Just as the term was drawing to a close, word came of the death of their aunt and girls returned to Yorkshire. Shortly thereafter, M. Heger wrote suggesting one or both return to Brussels to teach in the school, a proposal Charlotte accepted with alacrity.

The 1842-1844 Brussels interlude proved an extremely strong influence on Charlotte Brontë's development. While there, she matured, both chronologically and emotionally, broadened her experiences and understanding, and developed critical skills in expression. But there was much more, and many modern Brontë scholars believe those two years or so in Brussels represented a defining influence on the writer that Charlotte Brontë would become. For it was here that she first experienced love—love that turned out to be love for a married man. To Charlotte, M. Heger represented much more than a charismatic teacher; however, her infatuation with him was not reciprocated.

Returning to Haworth, Charlotte found a dispiriting set of circumstances. Her father's eyesight was failing rapidly. Her brother had failed in a number of different positions and his life was spiraling downward in alcohol and opium. The school the three Brontë girls had hoped to start died on the vine when newspaper advertisements elicited not a single response. Charlotte found her respite in writing poetry and, on discovering that her sisters Emily and Anne were similarly engaged, she suggested jointly publishing a volume of their poetry. With some difficulty, they found a publisher, but the terms required that the authors pay in advance the full cost of publication (today such a publishing house is called a "vanity press"). They paid with part of the inheritance from their aunt. In view of the prevailing bias against women writers, the girls decided on masculine-sounding pseudonyms: Currer for Charlotte, Ellis for Emily, and Acton for Anne, all with the surname of Bell.

In May 1846, *Poems* by Currer, Ellis, and Acton Bell, a volume of 165 pages, was released. The reviews were moderately favorable but the venture turned out to be anything but a success commercially: a grand total of two copies were sold! Such an experience might discourage some, but within a year of the release of *Poems*, Charlotte wrote a potential publisher that the Bells "are now preparing for the Press a work of fiction—consisting of three distinct and unconnected tales which may be published either together as a work of 3 vols of the ordinary novel-size, or published as single vols." The novel Charlotte was writing, entitled *The Professor*, tells of a young man who moves to Brussels as a schoolteacher and falls in love with an Anglo-Swiss pupil. Emily's novel was *Wuthering Heights*, set in the wild and desolate Yorkshire moors so familiar to the Brontës, it would become a classic of doomed love, unspeakable cruelty, and abject betrayal. Anne's work, *Agnes Grey*, told a story of the heart-rending trials of a governess.

Completed in July 1846, the novels were packaged under the Bell pseudonyms and begun on a weary round of publishers that would not end until a year later, and even then any victory was incomplete. A publishing house expressed interest in Emily's and Anne's novels—but only if the authors would again bear the costs—and not in Charlotte's under any circumstances. Now with her novel standing alone, Charlotte sent it to many more publishers but there were no takers. Years later, after Charlotte was a famous (and dead) author, *The Professor* would finally be published.

Just as the constant round of rejections began to dim Charlotte's enthusiasm, there came a faint ray of hope from the last publisher to whom she had sent *The Professor*, Smith, Elder & Co. of London. George Smith, the young owner of this small but good publishing house, can rightfully claim to be responsible for discovering Charlotte Brontë. Although he declined to publish the novel, his letter contained an extensive and useful critique and, moreover, indicated an interest in seeing something else she might write.

Charlotte was already well along with another novel, which she finished while nursing her father as he recovered from eye surgery. Again under the name of Currer Bell, the novel told the story of an orphaned girl named Jane who, after being sent to a miserably cruel school (modeled on the Cowan Bridge School Charlotte held responsible for death of her two elder sisters), becomes governess to the daughter of a (presumably) widowed and darkly fascinating but troubled man. Small and plain in appearance but intelligent, spirited, and capable, Jane falls in love with her charge's father. However, she then learns the man has an insane wife incarcerated in the attic. Jane flees and is taken in by a minister who, after she has recovered her emotional health, asks her to marry him and go to India as a missionary. But an eerie call brings Jane back to the house of her former lover for one last look, and she discovers that it has been burned to the ground by a fire that killed the mad wife and blinded the master. The lovers are reunited and together they find happiness. The novel, with certain obvious autobiographical elements, was entitled *Jane Eyre* and it became one of the enduring classics of English literature. At its publication in October 1847, having been rushed into print ahead of Emily's and Anne's novels sitting at another publisher, it was hugely popular and it has never been out of print since.

The critics were not entirely unanimous in their approbation of *Jane Eyre*. Several commented on the novel's "coarseness," meaning a hint of improper behavior (although by 20th century standards it was extremely mild). In response, Charlotte inserted a preface in the second edition in which she wrote: "Conventionality is not morality. Self-righteousness is not religion." The unfavorable reviews notwithstanding, the public was enthralled with the work—and has remained so, as succeeding generations have re-discovered it. Everyone in London wondered about the identity of this astonishing author, Currer Bell. The Brontë sisters maintained their anonymity assiduously until a rumor (probably initiated by an unscrupulous publisher) surfaced that Currer, Ellis, and Acton Bell were actually one person. Incensed, they hurried to London and presented themselves to Smith, Elder & Co., exposing their true identities.

As 1847 merged into 1848, it seemed that the trials of the Brontë family were over. The success of *Jane Eyre* was matched, or nearly so, by Emily's and Anne's novels and their father's eyesight had been restored by surgery. Then, over the span of eight months beginning in late September 1848, all three of Charlotte's remaining siblings died of fulminate tuberculosis. Branwell was the first to go and his death at age 29, while not exactly unexpected in view of his alcohol and opium addiction, caused Charlotte much anguish. The relationship between sister and brother, only a year apart in age, had been a complex amalgam of love, cooperation, and rivalry during childhood; by the time of his death, she was left only with a bitter sadness at his dissipated gifts and wasted opportunities. Emily and Anne in turn developed respiratory symptoms, which progressed rapidly and caused their deaths at 30 and 29, respectively. And so, by the end of May 1849, Charlotte found herself alone and, as she put it in a letter to her publisher, "Papa has now me only – the weakest – puniest – least promising of his six children."

Seared by tragedy and now solely responsible for her demanding father, Charlotte found redemption in writing. She completed *Shirley*, a novel set in the west of Yorkshire at the time of labor unrest in the early 19th century. She also occupied herself with cementing the literary legacies of her departed sisters, and in 1850 published a new one-volume edition of *Wuthering Heights* and *Agnes Grey* with a preface containing extensive biographical information. A new novel, *Villette*, set in Brussels and based largely on her experiences there, appeared in 1853. As the identity of Currer Bell gradually became known, Charlotte found herself faced with many accompaniments of fame—invitations to parties, meeting famous people, sitting for portraits, and answering correspondence—and most of them were ordeals for her. And, of course, there was her primary responsibility of caring for her aging father.

When Charlotte's identity was revealed, many expressed wonder that such a plain-appearing woman could be the source of such lyrical, romantic writing. But Charlotte Brontë's life had not been devoid of romance. She undoubtedly was in love with Constantin Heger, her teacher in Brussels, and probably also with George Smith, her publisher, although in both cases it was unrequited. She had received at least three marriage proposals, all of which she declined. Just as she was probably resigning herself to spinsterhood, there came another proposal. Arthur Bell Nicholls had a familiar background—born in Northern Ireland, well educated (in his case at Trinity College, Dublin), and ordained in the Anglican Church. He had served as curate (i.e., assistant) to Charlotte's father for seven years and surprisingly in December 1852 he asked Charlotte to marry him. Her reaction was guardedly positive but her father was strongly opposed and, ever the obedient daughter, Charlotte declined the offer. Nichols left Haworth, but he wrote many letters imploring her to reconsider. Finally, she began answering his letters and eventually they met to work things out. By this time, The Reverend Mr. Brontë's opposition had softened and he consented if Nicholls would agree to return as his curate and the couple would live in the parsonage. The wedding took place on June 29, 1854 in Haworth and the couple left for a month-long honeymoon in Ireland.

Illness and Death

Returning home at the beginning of August, Charlotte was supremely happy and her letters reflected a new degree of contentment and equanimity. Moreover, she seemed in better health than had been the case in years, writing to a friend "It is long since I have known such comparative immunity from headache, sickness, and indigestion as during the past three months." Shortly after the new year, however, there was a clear change. On January 19, she wrote to Ellen Nussey that all had been well until ten days earlier when "the stomach seemed quite suddenly to lose its tone, indigestion and continual faint sickness has been my portion ever since." She cautioned against any conjecture, "for it is too soon yet though I certainly never before felt as I have done lately." Thus, about the middle of January, Charlotte was seized with severe and unrelenting nausea and nearly continuous vomiting, followed shortly by recurring faintness. She had no interest in food at all and, when forced to consume something, she immediately vomited. The condition persisted and, according to one of the household employees, "a wren would have starved on what she ate during those last six weeks."

After a month or so of vomiting, Charlotte's condition had caused enough alarm that she acceded to her husband's urging that a physician be called. According to an early biographer, the doctor "assigned a natural cause for her miserable indisposition and said it would pass," something generally interpreted as indicating the problem was felt to be related to early pregnancy. However, her symptoms did not relent, and in fact became worse. She weakened gradually and became emaciated, spending more and more of her time in bed. On February 17, she made her will, rescinding the pre-nuptial agreement by which, if she died without children, her estate would pass to her father rather than her husband; in the will she left everything to her beloved Arthur. Toward the end, Charlotte became delirious and actually begged for food. In the early hours of March 31, while her husband was praying God to spare her, she became lucid and said "Oh! I am not going to die, am I? He will not separate us, we have been so happy." But Charlotte Brontë Nicholls—as she had been signing her letters—was dead, three weeks before her 39th birthday. Following a funeral in the church where she had been married and her father had served as rector for 35 years, Charlotte Brontë was buried in the family vault, joining her mother and four siblings (Anne having been buried at the seaside town where she had gone in hopes a visit to the beach would restore her precarious health).

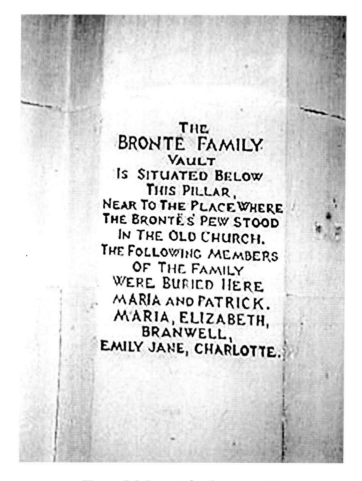

Figure 5.2 Brontë family memorial,
Church of Saint Michael and All Angels, Haworth, Yorkshire
(Courtesy of Scott McElwain)

Her husband kept his promise to live in the parsonage and care for his father-in-law until the latter died in 1861, aged 85 and outliving by many years his wife and children. Although Arthur Bell Nicholls had carried virtually the full load of parish work for a number of years, he was not particularly popular with the parishioners and therefore he did not receive the permanent appointment as rector of the Haworth church. So he returned to his native Ireland, taking with him, as was his right according to his late wife's will, as much of Charlotte Brontë's personal and literary possessions as he could keep from the hands of souvenir hunters. Later, he remarried and lived until the age of 88, all the while serving as a quiet and dignified custodian of his many important Brontë relics.

Immediately after Charlotte's death a number of newspaper articles speculated about her life history. Some of them were wildly inaccurate and a few were even lurid. To protect her reputation, her father invited Elizabeth Gaskell to write a biography. In many ways Mrs. Gaskell, the wife of a Unitarian minister, was ideally suited to the task. Herself a successful novelist and Charlotte's friend for the last several years of her life, she was given access to Charlotte's voluminous correspondence, notably over 300 letters to Ellen Nussey, and she interviewed all the people who played important roles. She applied herself with great energy and *The Life of Charlotte Brontë*, appeared within two years of its subject's death. The Gaskell biography painted Charlotte as a tragic figure, almost a martyr, caught in a web of terrible circumstances, none of them of her own doing. Virtually ignoring her intellectual qualities, independent spirit, and sometimes cynical nature, it gave rise to a "Charlotte Brontë myth" that has persisted to the present. For example, Mrs. Gaskell interviewed M. Heger and was shown Charlotte's love letters to him, but she chose to ignore the matter entirely. There have been many subsequent biographies of Charlotte Brontë, extending virtually to the present day, that have presenting contrasting views, but all stand to some extent in the shadow of Mrs. Gaskell's work simply because it was the first and was based so heavily—if selectively—on Charlotte's own words.

The Gaskell biography also emphasized Charlotte's struggle against the discrimination and inequities faced by women in mid-19th century England. As a result of this portrayal, she would later come to be regarded as one of the pioneers of feminism, earning her a devoted and fervent following that persists to this day. Charlotte's place as an icon of the feminist movement is deserved, notwithstanding her meek subservience to her father, and requires no more eloquent proof than the words she put in Jane Eyre's mouth:

> *Women are supposed to be very calm generally: but women feel just as men feel; they need exercise for their faculties, and a field for their efforts as much as their brothers do; they suffer from too rigid a restraint, too absolute a stagnation, precisely as men would suffer; and it is narrow-minded in their more privileged fellow-creatures to say that they ought to confine themselves to making puddings and knitting stockings, to playing on the piano and embroidering bags. It is thoughtless to condemn them, or laugh at them, if they seek to do more or learn more than custom has pronounced necessary for their sex.*

The cause of Charlotte Brontë's death has been the subject of much attention and no little controversy. In the main, three causes have been proposed and debated: typhoid, tuberculosis, and *hyperemesis gravidarum* (a Latin term meaning severe and excessive vomiting of pregnancy). Typhoid was common in Haworth in the mid-19th century, due to unsanitary living and a contaminated water supply. Moreover, an elderly domestic employee of the Brontë household had died a few weeks before Charlotte and the cause was felt to be typhoid. However, although typhoid is an infection of the alimentary tract, it manifests itself almost entirely as diarrhea and vomiting is not a common symptom. There is no indication in any of the records that Charlotte had diarrhea, but there is abundant evidence that vomiting was her major if not her sole complaint. Thus, while typhoid represents a plausible explanation, it probably is the least likely and none of the several physicians who have analyzed the case over the years have favored it.

Tuberculosis has much in its favor as a diagnosis. It was, of course, rampant in the Brontë family, almost surely the cause of death of all five of Charlotte's siblings and quite likely of her mother as well. Virtually everyone in 19th-century Europe came in contact with the organism that causes tuberculosis. Many were able to contain the infection and suffer little or no adverse effects on their health, but in a substantial proportion, probably as much as a quarter, the body defense mechanisms proved inadequate and clinical disease ensued. Called at the time "consumption," this was usually a condition with a slowly progressive downhill course, most often involving the lungs but sometimes affecting other organs. Occasionally, it would follow a much more acute course (as seemed to be the case with the five Bonté children), due presumably to impaired defenses in the affected individual or a particularly virulent strain of infecting organism.

Charlotte Brontë's death certificate listed as the cause of her death "pthisis," Greek for consumption. She undoubtedly had the disease and some of her symptoms, notably diminished appetite and weight loss, are consistent with it. Nevertheless, several circumstances argue against it as causing her death. Chief among these inconsistencies is the overwhelming presence of severe and persistent vomiting, which is certainly not common with tuberculosis. Further, there is no indication that cough or other pulmonary symptoms were prominent. Thus, the majority opinion among medical experts familiar with the case seems not to favor tuberculosis as the proximate cause of her death.

This leaves *hyperemesis gravidarum*, severe and excessive vomiting related to pregnancy. Some degree of nausea, often accompanied by vomiting, is a near-universal complaint in early pregnancy. Rarely, the symptoms may be so severe and prolonged as to impair health; not only is the intake of fluids and nutrients curtailed and even eliminated, but there is also excessive loss through regurgitation. If vomiting is severe and prolonged, the body loses fluids and electrolytes and excessive acid accumulates in the blood because of breakdown of body tissues—in other words, the net effect is that of starvation.

Central to the issue of whether or not this caused her death is the question of whether Charlotte Brontë was actually pregnant because, if she were not pregnant, hyperemesis obviously could not have been the cause of death. The evidence seems clear, from both her letters and the Gaskell biography, that Charlotte believed herself to be with child. Moreover, this aspect was never disputed by her father or her husband, the two people closest to her during her final illness. There were no reliable tests to confirm pregnancy in the 1850s. She was seen once or twice by a physician but it seems unlikely that an appropriate examination was done to assess for pregnancy. Menstrual history (i.e., whether or not menstruation continued) would be helpful, but there is no mention of the matter, perhaps reflecting sensitivities of the Victorian age.

The case has been examined from a medical perspective on a number of occasions and a consensus seems be developing among gynecologists and other physicians that she died from dehydration, exhaustion, imbalance of sodium and other electrolytes, and loss of nutrients, all because of severe, intractable vomiting associated with early pregnancy—in other words, *hyperemesis gravidarum*. This opinion is not quite unanimous and a forceful and articulate minority position posits other causes, but hyperemesis clearly seems to be the majority opinion.

Medical Perspectives

Nausea and vomiting are very common complaints during early pregnancy. At least three-quarters of pregnant women experience some degree of nausea and most of these vomit occasionally. The symptoms often occur when the stomach is empty and thus are usually most evident on arising; hence the common name "morning sickness." However, nausea with or without vomiting can occur throughout the day. The onset comes within three or four weeks of conception—for many women morning sickness provides the first indication they might be pregnant—and the symptoms typically subside by the end of the first third of gestation, although occasionally they may persist until later in pregnancy. Thus, pregnancy nausea is a common condition, so common as to be considered virtually a normal concomitant of gestation, and in all but the most severe forms it does not carry any increased risk of problems for either mother or child. In fact, some research has even found that pregnant women who experience nausea actually tend to have better outcomes than those who do not.

The reason for this common symptom of early pregnancy is not known, although there have been many theories proposed. About a hundred years ago, in the wake of the revolutionary concepts of psychoanalysis put forth by Sigmund Freud, many conditions and illnesses were suspected of being based on psychological or emotional factors. The psychoanalytic explanation of vomiting during early pregnancy is that it represents a subconscious attempt on the part of a neurotic woman, ambivalent about having a child, to rid herself of the pregnancy. While some still hold to this psychological explanation, the majority opinion seems to have swung over the past few decades toward a primary biological cause, perhaps with (as really is true with all biological states, conditions, and illnesses in the human) some over-lay of psychological or emotional factors.

The most popular candidate as a biological cause of nausea and vomiting of pregnancy is the hormone chorionic gonadotrophin (CG). CG is the quin-tessential pregnancy hormone and all modern pregnancy tests represent methods of detecting it. Produced by the conceptus beginning a few days after fertilization of the ovum, the hormone is secreted into blood and trans-ported to the ovary where it stimulates that organ to continue producing estrogen and progesterone, essential hormones for the maintenance of preg-nancy and for the development of the fetus and placenta. Thus, CG is essen-tial to the health of a pregnancy for without it estrogen and progesterone levels will fall in a few days and the products of conception will be lost with what is commonly termed "miscarriage."

CG production increases rapidly in the first few days and weeks after con-ception, its level in blood normally doubling every two or three days during this phase. Blood levels peak some 7-9 weeks after conception (9-11 weeks after the last menstruation). By this time, the early placenta has formed suf-ficiently to begin producing estrogen and progesterone on its own, so the need for CG lessens and its levels begin to fall. By the end of the third or fourth month, the amount of CG in blood is only about one-fifth what it was at its peak, and it persists at this level for the remainder of pregnancy.

The evidence that CG is responsible for nausea and vomiting of pregnancy is circumstantial, resting mainly on two observations. First, the stage of pregnancy when the symptom is most marked corresponds quite closely with the time when blood CG levels are highest. Second, nausea and vom-iting seem to be more prevalent and/or more severe in pregnancies associ-ated with high CG levels. One such condition is where there is more than one fetus (e.g., twins or triplets) and another is an abnormal pregnancy in which the placenta overgrows and there is no fetus (called trophoblastic dis-ease). Other hormones may be involved as well; for example, progesterone causes relaxation of certain types of muscle such as that lining the gastrointestinal tract, and progesterone is abundant during pregnancy. Psychological and emotional factors may also be a factor, although current thinking regards any such role as probably secondary to a biological basis.

Nausea and vomiting of early pregnancy are, as noted previously, so common as to be regarded almost as a normal concomitant of gestation. In the vast majority of instances, it is basically that—a little troublesome, perhaps, but self-limited and essentially part and parcel of having a baby, with no cause for concern or specific treatment. However, there exists a rare condition known by it Latin name, *hyperemesis gravidarum*, which is assumed to represent the far end of the spectrum. A specific definition of this condition is lacking, but the diagnosis is usually based on the following:

- severe and unrelenting vomiting several times each day, without any evidence of other coincidental diseases;
- physical evidence of dehydration such as dry membranes and wrinkled skin;
- laboratory findings of electrolyte imbalance and acid-base disturbances in the blood;
- significant weight loss (i.e., at least five per cent of pre-pregnancy body weight).

Hyperemesis gravidarum can be an extremely serious problem, particularly if not treated adequately; in addition to extensive loss of fluids and nutrients, the gastro-intestinal tract can be injured from violent retching and nutritional inadequacies can lead to neurologic problems. Before the modern age of medicine, the diagnosis carried a definite risk of death. For example there were four deaths among 65 women with hyperemesis hospitalized at the Boston Lying In Hospital in 1930-1935.

Treatment of nausea and vomiting of early pregnancy will depend on the severity of the symptoms. If, as is usually the case, there is only mild queasiness in the morning, with two or three episodes of vomiting over a week, all that will be necessary is small frequent feedings (to keep the stomach from becoming empty) of bland foods (such as soups or toast or crackers), along with avoiding any foods or other substances (such as iron or vitamin tablets) that upset the stomach. Ginger and acupuncture have been shown, in credible scientific studies, to be helpful. With more severe symptoms, drug treatment may need to be considered. A number of drugs, called anti-emetics, suppress the brain centers involved in vomiting and are at least partially effective in pregnancy-associated vomiting. Such drugs used to be used commonly but a more conservative attitude has developed because of apprehensions about congenital defects in the developing fetus. None of the drugs used for pregnancy nausea has been shown in scientific studies to do this, but the fear persists. A drug used widely for this purpose was withdrawn by the manufacturer a decade ago because of a rash of liability suits alleging the drug caused fetal malformations. The scientific evidence against any such relationship was overwhelming and the company never lost any of the suits. However, the cost of defending against them became too great compared with the drug's market.

A diagnosis of hyperemesis (e.g., a woman with severe and repeated vomiting who has lost eight pounds from her pre-pregnant weight of 120 pounds) should be a signal for more aggressive treatment. Anti-emetic drugs are indicated. Intravenous administration of fluids and electrolytes to replace losses is needed and this usually means hospitalization. Adequate fluids and electrolytes can be given intravenously but the number of calories that can be administered by this route is limited. Therefore, in the very rare instance in which a woman cannot take in anything orally for several weeks, it may be necessary to administer concentrated solutions of nutrients through a catheter placed in a large central blood vessel or a tube in the intestinal tract.

The consensus of opinion is that Charlotte Brontë was early in pregnancy and died of *hyperemesis gravidarum*. Assuming this to be correct, what would have happened if she were alive today? Unequivocally, she would not have died. An accurate diagnosis would be made, first by a pregnancy test and then by blood studies to exclude any underlying medical illness and to characterize her state with respect to fluid and electrolyte balance. She would be hospitalized and given anti-emetic drugs and intravenous fluids to replace her losses. With treatment that today is quite routine, she would have lived many years and presumably would have written many more novels. And she would have had a child, perhaps to carry on the remarkable Brontë legacy.

SOURCES

Fraser Rebecca. *The Brontës: Charlotte Brontë and Her Family.* Crown Publishers, New York. 1988.

Gaskell Elizabeth. *The Life of Charlotte Brontë.* First published 1857. Penguin Books. London and New York, 1997. Edited with introduction and notes by Elisabeth Jay.

Gordon Lyndall. *Charlotte Brontë*: A Passionate Life. Norton. New York and London. 1994.

Sellars Jane. *The British Library Writer's Lives: Charlotte Brontë.* Oxford University Press. New York. 1997

Fitzgerald JA. Death of elderly primigravida in early pregnancy; Charlotte Brontë. *N Y State J Med* 1979;79:196-9.

Gallagher HW. Charlotte Brontë: a surgeon's assessment. *Brontë Society Transactions* 1985;18:363-70.

Rhodes P. A medical appraisal of the Brontës. *Brontë Society Transactions* 1972;10:101-9.

Weiss G. The death of Charlotte Brontë. *Obstet Gynecol* 1991;78:705-8

CHAPTER 6
STEPHEN CRANE AND TUBERCULOSIS

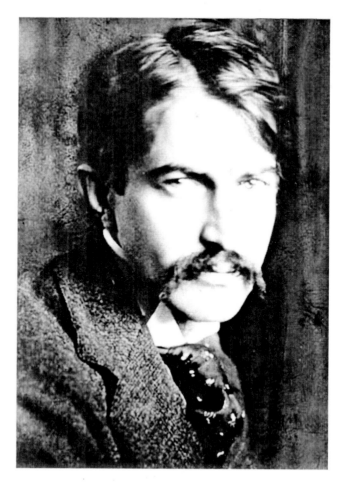

Figure 6.1 Stephen Crane (The Granger Collection, New York)

He was only 24 years old and lacked any experience in war or military matters when he produced his monumentally successful novel about the Civil War, *The Red Badge of Courage*. Stephen Crane pioneered a new style of writing that combined the gritty reality of ordinary people and their often bleak experiences with vivid imagery and symbolism, a style that produced lasting influences on fiction writing and made him an icon of modern literature. Contemporaries such as Joseph Conrad and Henry James and successors such as Ezra Pound and Ernest Hemingway, most of them better known than Crane today, acknowledged their debts to him. Crane's literary output—novels, short stories, poems, war reports, and newspaper articles, and other assorted writings—runs to ten volumes and is as remarkable for its versatility as for its volume. He died in 1900, at the age of only 28, of pulmonary tuberculosis, a disease that at the time was the principal scourge of the Western world. Today, tuberculosis has been largely contained in developed countries, mainly by improved living conditions and specific antibiotic therapy, but it remains a serious threat in the developing world.

Biography

On November 1, 1871, in Newark, New Jersey, a son was born to The Reverend and Mrs. Jonathan Townley Crane. It was the couple's 14th and last child; the four immediately preceding had each died in infancy, so this last child, given the name Stephen, had siblings ranging in age from 21 down to 8. Methodism ran in the family, for The Reverend Crane was a Methodist minister, as were his wife's father and uncle. Mrs. Crane, whose maiden name was Peck, was especially active in the Women's Christian Temperance Union and also worked in causes aimed at elevating the status of women.

Young Stephen's parents were occupied with their various activities and to a considerable extent the boy was raised by his older siblings. He was especially close to Agnes, 16 years his senior, who taught him to read and write when he was only three or four. Upbringing in the Crane household was strict, but The Reverend Mr. Crane was gentle and not lacking in a sense of humor and Stephen, although he would later rebel against most Christian tenets, always referred to his parents in kind and affectionate ways. They also provided an environment that probably influenced Stephen more than he realized. His father, who possessed a doctorate in divinity, wrote a great deal—religious tracts against tobacco, alcohol, opium, dancing, card-playing, and baseball; several books; and of course sermons—and his mother was always writing letters or preparing speeches. Thus, Stevie (as the family called him) was immersed from birth in a sea of words.

When Stephen was 6, the family moved to Port Jervis, New York, where The Reverend Dr. Crane became pastor of Drew Methodist Church. The rural, pastoral setting afforded opportunities to hunt, fish, camp, and ride horses, a delightful place for a boy to grow up, and Stephen always considered it home. Here he also began his formal schooling; although somewhat behind in this regard because of some childhood illnesses, the richness of his home education allowed him to catch up quickly. Unfortunately, Stephen's idyllic world ended abruptly, scarcely 2 years after the move to Port Jervis, when his father died suddenly. The Widow Crane and Stephen moved in with an older son who was just setting up a law practice in Port Jervis. Three years later, when Stephen was 11, they moved to Asbury Park, a resort town on the New Jersey coast 120 miles away, where Helen Crane soon became president of the local WCTU chapter. Daughter Agnes, now 27 and unmarried, joined them, securing a teaching position. Tragedy struck again a year later when Agnes died of meningitis; Stephen never wrote of it in later life but Agnes had been a comforting and steadying influence and her death undoubtedly left him with a painful void.

By this time, the 14-year old lad had found two interests that would remain with him: baseball and writing. In September 1885, he enrolled at Pennington Seminary, a school his father had helped to found, where the curriculum included literature, history, and English composition, along with strong emphasis on football and baseball. Stephen completed 2 years at Pennington, leaving midway through the third when he was accused unjustly of misbehavior. His preparation was apparently sufficient that a few months later he was able to enroll in Claverack College and Hudson River Institute in New York's Hudson River Valley.

Young Crane found the military discipline at Claverack to his liking and, of course, he did well in baseball. But his academic record was uneven at best. Probably as a reaction against his religious upbringing, he sought ways of flouting convention, among them a cigarette habit that would remain with him for the rest of his life. He did have an essay published in the school newspaper, his first signed publication. After a year and a half at Claverack, which he would later call the happiest time of his life, the family decided that Stephen should transfer to Lafayette College in Pennsylvania to study mining engineering. Stephen, by then nearly 19, submitted, but he expressed his unhappiness by seldom attending classes and his main activities centered on Delta Upsilon fraternity and baseball. By the end of the term he had failed five of his seven classes and his Lafayette career was over. In January 1891, he enrolled at Syracuse University, but again his main emphasis seems to have been on baseball, fraternity life, and defying school rules. He spent much of his time reading, including Tolstoy's massive novels *War and Peace* and *Anna Karenina*, and he honed his writing skills as his literary interests matured. But again it was one term and out.

When not in school, Stephen lived in Asbury Park with his brother, Townley, who was building a newspaper career. Townley published one paper, the *Newark Advertiser*, and ran an agency that supplied news items to New York papers and the Associated Press. During summers, Stephen worked for his brother, 19 years his senior, reporting on local news, particularly items related to the area's resort and vacation industry. Whatever of Stephen's items Townley chose to print appeared unsigned, but the experience was good for the budding writer.

His formal education over, Stephen went on an extended camping trip with some friends to the rugged woods of Sullivan County, New York, where he struck up conversations with local residents. Out of this experience came a number of short stories, some humorous but others rather dark. A few were published in the *New York Tribune*, this time with a by-line. About this same time, on August 17, 1891, he covered a lecture on an emerging style of writing called realism, defined as "the truthful treatment of commonplace material," even to the extent of including dialogue of colloquial speech. It was an epiphany for Crane, something he had sensed but had not comprehended so clearly. It would influence his subsequent fiction writing profoundly and in ways that would lead him ultimately to an iconic place in modern literature.

With summer coming to an end and vacationers leaving Asbury Park, the work Townley could give his brother diminished, so Stephen moved to the home of another brother, Edmund, in suburban Patterson, New Jersey. There was easy access to New York and the young writer began spending most of his time in The Bowery, a tawdry area of Manhattan full of saloons, brothels, dance halls, and cheap hotels. Sometimes he would go there for the day but other times he would stay over a night or two in one of the flophouses, getting to know the local population. He sought employment with all the New York papers, but none would hire one so young and inexperienced. When summer came again, he returned to Asbury Park to report on resort activities for Townley. In this, his 20th summer, he also fell in love, with a woman who was slightly older than he and was also married, albeit unhappily. The attraction was mutual, but Stephen failed in efforts to convince her to divorce her husband. He was crestfallen, but his productivity did not suffer. He wrote several more short stories for the Tribune and he began a novel based on his experiences in The Bowery.

In October 1892, Stephen moved back to Manhattan and to a shabby rooming house. It was the "Gay Nineties" and, living the bohemian life and consorting with the low lifes of New York City, he refined and revised his novel about a young prostitute. One publisher found it intriguing but too controversial, so Crane decided to publish it himself; his mother had just died and he used a small inheritance from her. It appeared in early 1993, under the title *Maggie: A Girl of the Streets*, for some reason Crane chose the pseudonym Johnston Smith. Sales were negligible but Stephen was not particularly discouraged. About this same time his interest turned to the Civil War, now 30 years past. He read a series of magazine articles about the conflict, finding them interesting but written in a sterile, emotionless manner, describing what the people involved did but not how they felt. Gradually, the idea for a novel took shape and he began planning a story about a young man who joins the Union Army full of patriotism and idealism, but soon becomes, first, discouraged by the dullness of Army routine and, then, appalled by the abject horror of war itself. As always, since he didn't own a typewriter, he wrote in longhand on yellow legal tablets. The book, originally entitled *Private Fleming, His Various Battles*, had begun to taken shape when Stephen moved back to live with his brother, Edmund.

Living with Edmund's family throughout the summer of 1893 proved an excellent setting for Stephen to work on his new novel. He often worked all night, writing and revising, and then slept until noon. By September, when he returned to New York City, the novel was in near-final draft form. During the same interval he wrote a number of newspaper articles and completed a set of poems (which he always called "lines"). The former were successful in bringing some money, but the latter proved more problematic, mainly because they were written in free verse style and non-rhyming poems were not well accepted at the time. Finally, a "progressive" publishing house agreed to publish the poems as a book called *The Black Raiders and Other Lines*. Meanwhile, Crane completed his Civil War novel, now entitled *The Red Badge of Courage, An Episode of the Civil War*. At the end of April 1894, he offered it to Samuel McClure, who had published material on the Civil War; McClure recognized the novel's value instantly but he was currently short of money, so he stalled, hoping his financial situation would improve. Stephen wrote some newspaper and magazine articles on various subjects, several of which received favorable notice, so he was beginning to develop a reputation as a writer.

After waiting 6 months, Crane had finally had enough of McClure's stalling. He took *The Red Badge of Courage* to the Bacheller Syndicate, which agreed immediately to syndicate the novel (i.e., publish it in abridged form serially in newspapers). The first installment appeared in December 1893 and eventually the series ran in 750 papers over the country. It was hugely successful and a publisher, The D. Appleton Company, expressed interest in publishing the book in its full form. Over the next year, Crane found several jobs to keep occupied. The most important of these came from Bacheller Syndicate itself. Seeing an opportunity to capitalize on the highly successful syndication, Batcheller commissioned Stephen to travel throughout the Midwest and South, with articles sent to the news agency at each stop. The tour lasted several months and included stops in St, Louis, Omaha, New Orleans, Galveston, and Mexico City. On Stephen's return, the book of poetry had just been published and, while critics were anything but enthusiastic about his "lines," he reveled in seeing his poetry in print. Further, in June, Crane finally received a contract from Appleton to publish *The Red Badge of Courage*. The terms were not very favorable from the author's perspective, but he signed anyway because he was interested in finally getting the book published. Later, he would learn that Appleton had sold publication rights to a British company without any provision for author royalty. The book became, if anything, more popular in Britain than in the United States and the English publisher wrote Crane "how pleased we are to be identified with your work," but none of it produced anything tangible to the author.

By the beginning of 1896, Stephen Crane was becoming known both at home and abroad and his main concern, expressed privately, was how he could sustain the momentum. Critics showered extravagant praise on his novel and Civil War veterans found his battle descriptions so vivid and realistic they had difficulty believing he had not been involved. In fact, he had never experienced war in any way and his military background was negligible, yet his incredible imagery seemed to capture the essence of combat. Most of his descriptions concerned the abject horror of battle, but some emphasized a poignant and less violent side. One example of the latter is a description of the aftermath of a battle, one from which Private Fleming had initially run away and then returned to:

> On the other side of the fire the youth observed an officer asleep, seated bolt upright, with his back against a tree. There was something perilous in his position. Badgered by dreams, perhaps, he swayed with little bounces and starts, like an old, toady-stricken grandfather in a chimney corner. Dust and stains were upon his face. His lower jaw hung down as if lacking strength to assume its normal position. He was the picture of an exhausted soldier after a feast of war.

Publishers, wishing to capitalize on Crane's fame, clamored for more of his writings. In relatively short order, he wrote a number of short stories and articles, including a series about famous Civil War battlefields; he prepared a somewhat sanitized revision of *Maggie*; and he completed another novel, *George's Mother*. These activities provided him, for the first and probably only time in his life, with adequate income. Then things began to unravel. While doing a series of feature articles on a vice-ridden area of New York City, he observed a prostitute he judged being treated unfairly by police, and he took up her cause. His testimony at her trial led to her acquittal, but then he went further by encouraging and supporting her civil action against the police department. In the process, he was roundly criticized throughout the country and his recent fame soured. He escaped by accepting an offer to go to Cuba to report on the recent uprising against Spanish rule, stopping on the way in Jacksonville, Florida. Here he met a woman who would become the major influence on the remainder of his life. She was Cora Stewart: sophisticated, well-read, six years his senior, twice married—and madam of a brothel called Hotel de Dream.

Shortly after meeting Cora, Stephen took passage on a tugboat bound for Cuba, sailing on New Year's Eve. The ship hit a sandbar shortly after departure, sustaining damage that led to its foundering in open sea. Following a harrowing 24 hours in which several crewmen drowned, Crane was eventually rescued. He returned to Jacksonville to write of his experience for the newspaper syndicate sponsoring his travel, followed by a fictionalized version, *The Open Boat*, that in more modern times would come to be regarded as a literary classic. His relationship with Cora deepened and, when the *New York Journal* engaged him to cover an impending war between Greece and Turkey, he convinced the paper to hire her to report the war from a woman's point of view. The couple sailed separately, Stephen stopping first in London where he was feted because of the popularity of *The Red Badge of Courage*, and then on to Greece. Here Crane would see war for the first time, and although the war lasted only a few weeks, he managed to send his paper at least 13 dispatches, all of them blending literary imagination with strict reporting.

Stephen and Cora decided against returning to America. He was popular in England, in contrast to the lingering animosity about his controversy with the New York City Police Department. Moreover, his finances had reverted to a precarious state, and creditors were harassing him. But the primary consideration was undoubtedly the nature of their relationship. Some sources suggested they had married but, even if true, it would have been illegal, for Cora was not divorced from her second husband. So they settled into a house in Surrey, a few miles outside London, as Mr. And Mrs. Stephen Crane, and a lifestyle that far exceeded their means.

Stephen continued writing, mainly short stories based on earlier travels through America, and English reviewers were generally much kinder than those in his native land. To stem a rising tide of debt, he flooded his American agent with articles, some good and some not, imploring him to seek larger and larger advances. As his financial woes were deepening, Stephen's frenetic writing turned almost frantic. However, it was at this time that he had the good fortune to meet Joseph Conrad, with whom he would form a literary association and friendship that would deepen and blossom over the next two years.

In April 1898, opportunity knocked. The U. S. battleship Maine had blown up in Havana harbor and a Spanish-American War seemed inevitable. Stephen sailed to New York and thence to Key West, Florida, with a commission to report for the *New York World*. It took a few weeks, but eventually the war came and Stephen got to Cuba in time to witness American marines landing at Guantanamo Bay on June 10. He covered all the important actions, including the charge of Roosevelt's Rough Riders up San Juan Hill, filing vivid accounts of each to his newspaper. He contracted malaria, causing him to return to America to recuperate. For reasons unclear, his job with the *New York World* ended, but he got a position with the *New York Journal* that took him first to Puerto Rico, where the war was now in its final stages, and then to Havana. Spain still controlled Havana and American correspondents were unwelcome, but Crane stayed there for some weeks, sending out many newspaper articles, a number of short stories, and enough poems for his second book of poetry, and he also started a novel. This burst of productivity was probably driven by continuing financial pressures, for the *New York Journal* had fired him for abusing his expense account. Curiously, he did not write Cora at all during this period, suggesting to some that he may have been involved with another woman. Cora, busy fending off creditors in England, managed to find a possible book contract for Stephen and wrote imploring him to come home. Eventually he did, arriving after a 9-month absence on January 11, 1899.

Nothing had changed. The rent on their house had not been paid for a year and local merchants were pressing for payment of long-overdue bills, yet the Cranes continued their extravagant lifestyle. A number of literati lived in the neighborhood, including Joseph Conrad, Henry James, H. G. Wells, and the renowned critic Edward Garnett, and the Cranes entertained them lavishly. Forced to move, the Cranes found Brede Place, a ramshackle, drafty house lacking any modern convenience but available to them under favorable terms. Their financial problems were formidable—Stephen, in his own words, continued to "borrow money from near every body in the world"— and bankruptcy was averted by the narrowest of margins. But money was not the most serious problem, for Stephen's health now showed clear signs of deterioration.

Illness and Death

A tendency for consumption (the term for tuberculosis for most of history) to run in families had long been recognized and until the infectious nature of the disease was established in the late 19th century, one theory held that it was hereditary. Of course, the familial predilection simply reflected close living conditions. In the case of the Crane family, there is really only one clear instance of tuberculosis, and it occurred before Stephen's birth. An aunt, the sister of Stephen's father, died "bleeding at the lungs" while living with the Cranes in 1867. As noted earlier, a number of Stephen's siblings died in infancy, but their deaths seem more likely due to the many childhood illness rampant at that time, rather than to tuberculosis. In essence, then, the Cranes seemed less "consumptive" than the average family of the time.

It is difficult to pin down the time Stephen first came in contact with the disease that would eventually kill him. He was a rather sickly child, afflicted with frequent colds, and his father's diary contained at least one reference to concern for the health of his youngest child. Although this could conceivably have reflected the onset of his chronic illness, such a possibility seems unlikely. As Stephen grew into adolescence and then adulthood, he reveled in the active, outdoor type of life, being especially fond of horseback riding, camping, hunting and fishing. In addition, his love of baseball, coupled with some apparent ability in the sport, argues against him having any significant degree of chronic disease at the time.

A likely possibility for the onset of his illness is the time in 1891 when he began living in The Bowery in order to experience the seamy side of life he was interested in writing about. New York City at the time had one of the world's highest rates of tuberculosis and nowhere was the disease more frequent than in the crowded and foul slums of Lower Manhattan. It would be rare indeed for one to spend any significant time there without encountering tuberculosis. Friends later recalled that Stephen's persistent, hacking cough seemed to begin at about this time, although that symptom could also have been due to his heavy cigarette smoking.

There is incontrovertible evidence of the diagnosis in the summer of 1898, during the interval between his two trips to Cuba covering the Spanish-American War. While in New York, he apparently traveled to Saranac Lake in the Adirondacks to see Dr. Edward Trudeau, a well-known specialist in lung disease, specifically tuberculosis. The only record of that visit is a letter dated September 16, 1898 from Dr. Trudeau to Cora, Stephen's common-law wife, in England:

*Your husband had a slight evidence of activity in the trouble
in his lungs when he came back this summer but it was not
serious and he improved steadily I understand since he came.
I have only examined once but he looked very well and told me
he was much better than last time I saw him.*

What Trudeau calls "activity" is a euphemism for consumption. However,
the ability to assess tuberculous activity accurately in 1898 was limited,
based on history, temperature, and findings on listening to the chest with a
stethoscope. X-rays had been discovered in 1896 but their use in diagnos-
ing chest conditions was well in the future. Thus, Trudeau's optimistic-
sounding letter was really based on limited information. One interesting
footnote is the indication that he had seen Crane previously; there is no
record of an earlier visit but the mention certainly implies the diagnosis had
been made before 1898.

By the time Stephen returned to New York on his way back to England from
Cuba, his physical deterioration was apparent to all who had known him.
One friend recorded: "He strikes me now as he did in early days as unwhole-
some physically—not a man of long life." No one seems to have used the
dreaded term consumption or its newer synonym, tuberculosis, but clearly
he was entering the terminal phase of the illness. Reaching England in early
January 1899, he threw himself feverishly into work, not driven by any artistic or creative urges but by the omnipresent financial pressures closing in
from all sides. He turned out short stories, feature articles, newspaper pieces
and anything else he had any hope of selling. Friends described him during
this time as spending nearly all day at his desk, smoking one cigarette after
another, sipping on a weak whiskey and soda, and writing continuously.
Some of what he wrote was quite good; perhaps the best was a very short
piece, *The Upturned Face,* about the burial of a soldier in the Spanish-
American War. But much of it was not at all good, and it soured his publishers and debased his reputation. He and Cora each wrote to his British
agent virtually every day—often more than once a day—asking, begging,
and sometimes demanding money—25 pounds for the wine dealer or 40
pounds for the butcher or 20 pounds so they might take a brief holiday.

Crane rarely complained about his health and seemed most of the time to
downplay any illness or incapacity. He spoke and wrote occasionally about
his "Cuban fever;" presumably a reference to malaria. It would be unusual
if he had not acquired malaria, since it was prevalent during his time in the
Caribbean, but this was not his major health problem. He seemed particularly intent on concealing the nature and severity of his illness from Cora and
on several occasions he cautioned friends about this point. Yet she knew as

well as he that he was failing rapidly. Nevertheless, both carried on the charade, she by suggesting he begin a popular novel to bring in much-needed money and he by actually making a good beginning on writing it.

The Cranes decided to throw a grand Christmas party, inviting a large number of their friends to their house for several days in late December 1899. Eventually, some 50 guests gathered at the drafty old Brede Place for three days of nonstop eating and drinking, most of them sleeping on cots rented from a local hospital. They participated in a play Stephen had written for the occasion, with music borrowed from Gilbert and Sullivan. The last evening, December 29, there was a grand ball. That night, after all had retired, Cora wakened H. G. Wells to tell him Stephen had suffered a "lung hemorrhage." It was probably not the first time he had coughed up blood. Wells rode a bicycle some seven miles in the late winter night to fetch a doctor. There was, of course, little anyone could do other than to hope he had no more hemorrhages. Stephen continued to work on novel he had begun about an Irish romance, but more and more he worked from bed. In early February, he attended a luncheon in his honor, and the guests were shocked by his wan appearance and subdued manner.

On March 31, Cora left for Paris to meet Stephen's niece who had been attending school in Switzerland. Shortly after her departure, Stephen began hemorrhaging and the cook, over Stephen's objections, telegraphed Cora in Paris. Cora wired the American embassy in London who dispatched a nurse and a physician to Brede Place. The author was now confined to bed, in hopes of forestalling any further lung hemorrhage. His condition seemed to stabilize and Cora over-optimistically reassured his agent and publishers that his contractual obligations would be fulfilled. Stephen was more realistic; he asked a visitor to read what he had written of his Irish romantic novel to see if he (the visitor) would like to finish it "since I will not be alive to do so."

By this time, Crane had come under the care of at least two "specialist" physicians: J. T. Maclagen (who had been sent originally by the American Embassy) and Mitchell Bruce. Their assessments, as reported by Cora, seem brazenly unrealistic. In mid-April, she wrote that the doctors were "hopeful" and "so encouraging that I am glad;" whether this reflected a cunning subterfuge to keep his agent and publishers paying, or simply naiveté, is unclear. One or both specialists recommended Stephen leave the unhealthful climate and environment of Brede Place and seek recuperation in a sanatorium. Badenweiler, in the Black Forest of Germany, was chosen. This would, of course, require money, and Cora (having recently taken over sole charge of Stephen's correspondence) undertook a nonstop fund-raising campaign. She wrote to every publisher, agent, or other business associate, past or present; to family and friends; and to all others she thought might be receptive to contributing. Included in this latter category were Lady Jennie Churchill, Joseph Pulitzer, J. P. Morgan, and Andrew Carnegie.

Cora's efforts were productive enough that Stephen and Cora, along with two nurses, a doctor, a valet, and Stephen's dog set out from Brede Place on the morning of May 5. They stopped at a hotel in Dover, to rest for the Channel crossing, and a steady stream of callers, including old friend Joseph Conrad, came to pay their respects. Stephen even found enough strength to dictate to Cora some of the still-unfinished Irish novel. On May 24 the entourage crossed the Channel to Calais, then took a carriage to Basel where they rested for several days at an expensive hotel. From there they traveled by carriage the final 30 miles to Badenweiler, taking rooms at the Villa Eberhardt.

Crane's doctor was Albert Frankel, head of the Hilaherin sanatorium and a well-qualified specialist in lung disease. He was sufficiently alarmed that he called in a consultant, a professor from Freiburg. Crane had fever, indicating the tuberculous process was especially active, and nothing could bring it down. Stephen continued dictating his Irish novel, now called *The O'Ruddy*, but he was becoming less and less coherent. Finally, on June 4, Cora finally accepted the inevitable and cabled William that his brother was dying. At 3 o'clock the next morning Stephen Crane died.

After embalming, the body was placed in a casket with a glass viewing panel and shipped to London and then across the Atlantic, accompanied by Cora. Stephen's deathbed wish was to be buried with his parents and, following a Methodist service at the Central Metropolitan Temple in New York, on June 28 he was laid to rest in the Crane family plot at the Evergreen Cemetery in Elizabeth, New Jersey.

Stephen had signed a new will just before leaving for the Black Forest. It named as his sole beneficiary "my dear wife Cora Crane," wording apparently chosen to protect her against any challenge to the legality of their relationship. In the event of Cora's death or remarriage, the estate was to be divided, half to Stephen's namesake nephew and half to brothers Edmund and William. The estate actually consisted of little other than enormous debts. Cora tried to fashion a writing career, finishing a few of Stephen's stories begun during his last several months, writing some of her own, and planning his biography, but it all came to little. She returned to England and then two years later came back to the United States. She even tried to return to her former "profession," opening a brothel in Jacksonville, and she married a man 15 years her junior. In 1910 she died and was buried under the name Cora Crane.

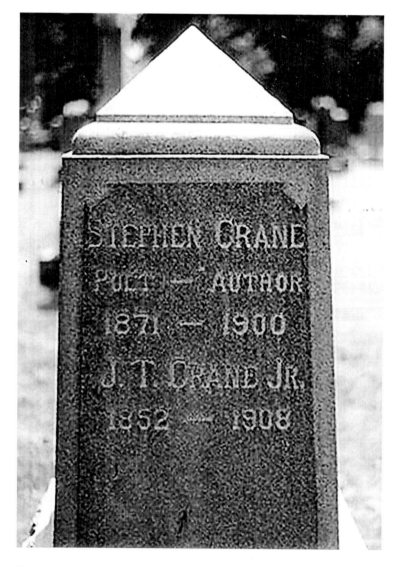

Figure 5.2 Tombstone of Stephen Crane and his brother, Townley, Evergreen Cemetery, Hillside, NJ (Courtesy of Kurt Lau)

Stephen Crane's literary legacy is more complicated than what he left in the way of tangible material. Twelve years after his death, Joseph Conrad bemoaned that no one remembered or cared about Crane, suggesting that "in fifty years some curious literary critic . . . will perhaps rediscover him." In reality, it didn't take nearly that long. The 1920s saw the beginning of a revival in interest in Crane's work. He became the subject of a number of doctoral dissertations and other critical analyses and his writings were

88

reprinted widely. There was an even greater peak of critical interest in the 1950s, and during that time *The Red Badge of Courage* was translated into a number of languages. As a result of all these activities, Crane came to be recognized as the main pioneer of "naturalism" in literature, one whose writings were basically realistic in portraying characters in their normal and usually bleak, dark circumstances, but with added flashes of imagery and symbolism. H. G. Wells described Crane's work as "the first expression of the opening mind of a new period, or, at least, the early emphatic phase of a new initiative." Among those who hailed his creative genius were his friends and associates Joseph Conrad, Henry James, and Willa Cather, but also later literary giants Ezra Pound, Robert Frost, and Ernest Hemingway who all acknowledged their debt to him.

A good summation of Crane comes from W. R. Irwin, Professor of English at the University of Iowa:

> *Crane spoke in a voice and with a manner which no one had used before him. He was like one of those musical phenomena whom humanity spawns occasionally—a child possessing the techniques of maturity. His vision was childlike in its unspoiled clarity, his writing essentially mature. He died early, leaving behind his instrument; and no one after him has ever been able to play it.*

Medical Perspectives

No disease has so much history and lore as has tuberculosis, its origins extending back into the dim recesses of human history. Evidence of it has been found in remains of prehistoric man and Hippocrates described the disease quite accurately. For most of history it was called consumption (or phthisis, the Greek word for consumption) because it seemed to "consume" the affected individual from within. The modern term tuberculosis was coined in 1839 because of the tubercles, masses of dense, fibrotic, inflammatory tissue, that characterize the disease.

A worldwide disease, tuberculosis was always common but its frequency seemed to grow to near-epidemic proportions in the 17th and 18th centuries, coinciding with the tendency of populations to aggregate into towns and cities. The process of urbanization and the incidence of clinical tuberculosis increased in lock-step manner as industrialization led to over-crowded living conditions, foul air and water, hunger, and poverty. Medical historian Roy Porter called tuberculosis "the single worst disease cultivated by monster cities." By the 19th century, a quarter of all adult deaths in Europe were due to it and the situation in American cities was little if any better. Tuberculosis was indeed, in the words of John Bunyan, "The captain of the men of death."

At the height of the tuberculosis epidemic, from perhaps the late 18th to the mid-19th century, the disease curiously acquired somewhat of a cachet—it was, after all, the Romantic Era—as a disease affecting particularly the upper classes and the literati. The image of consumptives was that of "beautiful people" and creative geniuses. For example, arguably the two most popular operas ever written, Verdi's *La Traviata* and Puccini's *La Bohème*, both concern women dying of consumption. The thin body, pale skin, and wan appearance characteristic of tuberculosis became desirable features, and so were produced by using face powder instead of rouge. But the association with privilege and creative genius was spurious. To be sure, tuberculosis afflicted people such as composers Frédéric Chopin and Carl Maria von Weber and poets John Keats and Percy Bysshe Shelley. However, it was, as it had always been, a disease predominately of the poor and downtrodden.

Historically, three causes of the disease were postulated: heredity, environment, and contagion. Each had a number of widely recognized associations in its support and arguments vacillated among the three putative explanations, with the consensus of medical authority sometimes favoring one and sometimes another. The matter was finally settled by the work of the German bacteriologist, Robert Koch, who on March 24, 1882 presented his results to the Berlin Physiological Society that established beyond any doubt the infectious nature of the disease. In one of the landmark events in the history of medicine, Koch proved tuberculosis due to a specific bacterium, subsequently named *Mycobcterium tuberculosis*. It was primarily this discovery that led to Koch's award of the Nobel Prize in Physiology or Medicine in 1905.

M. tuberculosis is an unusual organism in dividing much more slowly than other bacteria, accounting for the tendency of the disease to have a gradual and protracted course and one characterized by ups and downs in the clinical picture. The disease can be spread by several routes, but the most common and most dangerous is by droplets from the cough or expired air of someone whose lungs are infected. Usually, transmission comes with close contact over a long period and only rarely does a single sudden exposure lead to infection.

When an uninfected person comes in contact with the organism—and until the last several decades the vast majority did come into such contact sooner or later—one of two things happens. About 90% of the time, the newly infected individual's defense mechanisms isolate and contain the infection, most commonly in the lung itself. This state is called "latent tuberculosis" and it usually remains quiescent permanently (during which time there is no danger of transmission to others) and the individual never manifests any ill effects, although rarely resistance can break down and clinical or "active" disease ensue. The other outcome of primary infection, occurring in no more than 10% of primary exposures, is severe and widespread clinical disease, which without treatment can be rapidly fatal. Presumably, inadequate host defenses and/or exceptionally virulent organisms account for this unusual course.

Tuberculosis can affect nearly any organ or system in the body (especially bone, lymph nodes, genitourinary system, and brain), but the lung is the site of most common involvement and pulmonary tuberculosis is usually the most severe form, accounting for the vast majority of deaths. Organisms inhaled into the lung set up a primary infection that is usually walled off to become latent. Walled off, latent infection customarily remains quiescent but it can break down and become active. Presumably the determining factor in whether primary infection spreads or latent infection breaks down is resistance mediated through the host's immune system. Active disease in the lung causes tissue death, leading to formation of cavities often filled with a cheesy-like material; this process is called caseation and it causes a characteristic appearance on chest x-ray. Symptoms of active pulmonary tuberculosis include a hacking, persistent cough, often blood-stained; low grade fever and especially sweats at night; pallor; weight loss; and easy fatigability.

As the disease worsens, the infection may invade blood vessels in the lung, leading to bleeding. Usually bleeding in relatively minor, causing blood-streaked sputum, but if the vessel invaded happens to be a large one, the individual can actually bleed to death. Another and more common mechanism of death is pulmonary insufficiency due to widespread destruction of lung tissue. When the English poet, John Keats, died of tuberculosis at the age of only 24, autopsy revealed he had virtually no functional lung.

Around 1900, recognition of the infectious nature of the disease and understanding of its natural history led to public health measures aimed at containing it and improving the outcome of those infected. Both governments and non-governmental organizations became involved. Chief among the latter was the formation in 1904 of the National Association for the Study and Prevention of Tuberculosis, the first voluntary health organization dedicated to a single disease (and the predecessor of many such bodies). Composed mainly of lay people but with a strong medical involvement and direction as well, this organization conducted public education campaigns about tuberculosis, educated professionals, and sponsored medical care and assistance to families whose members had it. It became very efficient in raising money through the sales of "Christmas seals," placed on letters and cards at Christmastime, and its symbol, the red Lorraine cross, was ubiquitous. As it became clear that tuberculosis was under control, at least in the United States and other developed countries, the organization broadened its scope to include other lung diseases such as asthma, allergies, emphysema, cancer, and smoking-related conditions. Reflecting these shifts in emphasis are the organization's name changes, to the National Tuberculosis and Respiratory Disease Association in 1968 and finally to the American Lung Association in 1973.

Generally, the public health initiatives of governmental and non-governmental bodies fell into three main categories: public education, identifying new cases (e.g., by mass chest x-ray screening programs), and establishing sanatoria. The last of these, residential treatment facilities for tuberculous established throughout United States and Western Europe in the early 20th century, isolated infective patients and provided the only "treatments" known at the time to be helpful: good food, clean air, and healthful activities. In retrospect, questions have been raised about the efficacy of sanatoria (e.g., more than two-third of patients died within 5 years of admission), but sanatoria did represent one of the public health measures—others were enhanced public and professional education efforts, improved screening and case-finding, and a general improvement in living conditions—associated temporally with substantial decline in both incidence and mortality from tuberculosis. For example, mortality rates from the disease in Western European countries over the century from 1850 to 1950 fell from 300-500 per 100,000 population to as low as 50-100.

The first half of the 20th century saw remarkable success in immunizing against many different infections, leading to concerted efforts to develop a vaccine against tuberculosis. In spite of extensive study, these efforts proved disappointing; Robert Koch, who had established the bacterial nature of tuberculosis and several other diseases, failed miserably in efforts to produce a vaccine. There was one exception to the litany of failure, but even that has had a somewhat checkered career. Two French researchers, Calmette and Guérin, in the 1920s developed a vaccine using a weakened strain of the tubercle bacillus that affects cows. Called BCG after the discoverers, it proved effective in inducing immunity but its use has been controversial, not least because of an accident or two in which a dangerous form of the virus was used inadvertently. BCG was never used much in the United States or Western Europe, except for France, and at present it is advised only in areas of very high prevalence.

But the major development in tuberculosis control was a pharmacological one, the discovery of specific, effective drugs directed against the causative organism that represented the "magic bullet" envisioned by Paul Ehrlich a half-century earlier. Soon after its discovery, streptomycin, an antibiotic made by soil fungi, was seen to possess activity against M. tuberculosis and, in a landmark study conducted in Britain between 1946 and 1948, its efficacy in treating the disease was proven conclusively. (The study was also important in another way, for it represented the first randomized controlled trial of a medical treatment.) With effective antibiotic treatment, patients could be made non-infective quickly and could also anticipate arrest of their disease. Thus, beginning in about 1950, the apparatus built up over the preceding century—population screening programs using skin tests and chest x-rays, isolation of suspected cases, sanatorium treatment—no longer seemed necessary and was allowed to fade away.

Streptomycin proved effective in tuberculosis but it soon became clear that there were significant side effects and that bacteria tended to develop resistance to the agent. Other drugs were developed, particularly isoniazid, which became and has remained the primary therapeutic weapon. Development of drug resistance is always problematic because, even if only a small fraction of a type of bacteria is resistant to an antibiotic, that small fraction will survive and reproduce, soon becoming the predominant population of organisms. Resistance can usually be circumvented by employing a combination of drugs, since bacteria resistant to one agent are usually susceptible to a different one. For example, some 7% of initial infections are resistant to isoniazid but only 1% to isoniazid combined with another drug, rifampin. The most common approach today is to treat active cases with four drugs, isonizid, rifampin, pyrazinamide, and either streptomycin or ethambutol. In persons without evidence of disease but whose tuberculosis skin test has turned from negative to positive (meaning he or she has come in contact with the organism and may or may not have active disease), the recommended treatment is isoniazid for 9-12 months.

During the last 50 or 60 years, due mainly to drug therapy, both incidence and outcome of tuberculosis have improved dramatically, at least in developed countries. In the United States, for example, the number of new cases annually has fallen from nearly 80,000 in 1955 to 14,000 in 2005, and deaths have gone from 15,000 to 660 over the same period. Data demonstrating the effectiveness of drug treatment of tuberculosis are illustrated in the slide below, in which it is also apparent that deaths have fallen more steeply than cases.

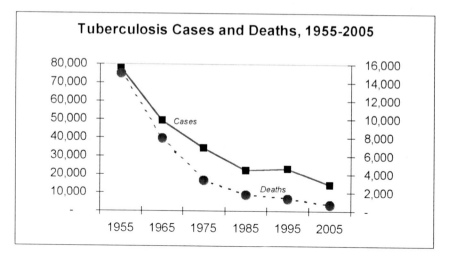

The worldwide situation is not nearly as sanguine as it is in developed countries like the United States and Western Europe. The World Health Organization reports that each year sees 9-10 million new cases and 2 million deaths. Even more concerning is the American Lung Association's estimate that between now and 2020, 1 billion people worldwide will be infected, 150 million will be come clinically ill, and 36 million will die. The two areas of the world with the greatest problem are Africa (particularly the sub-Saharan portion) and Southeast Asia. Three factors seem to be chiefly responsible for the ominous picture in these geographic areas: (1) over-crowded and poor living conditions and inadequate health care (just as have always been the case), (2) immunologic deficiency such as that with AIDS (often tuberculosis is the first manifestation of infection with the immunodeficiency virus), and (3) drug resistance, including resistance to multiple agents.

SOURCES

Davis Linda H. *Badge of Courage: The Life of Stephen Crane*. Houghton Mifflin. New York. 1998.

Lukes Bonnie L. *Soldier's Courage: The Story of Stephen Crane*. Morgan Reynolds. Greenboro NC. 2002

Bloom Harold. *Blooms Modern Critical Views: Stephen Crane*. Infobase. New York. 2007.

Stallman RW. *Stephen Crane: A Critical Bibliography*. Iowa State University Press. Ames IA. 1972

www.lungusa.org. Accessed March 27, 2008

CHAPTER 7
RUDOLPH VALENTINO AND PEPTIC UCLER

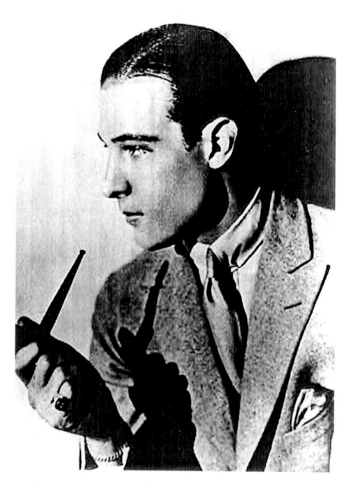

Figure 7.1 Rudolph Valentino (Library of Congress)

Valentino, the first and arguably the greatest movie celebrity, influenced 20th century culture in ways extending far beyond his brief film career. He brought to the movie screen a steamy eroticism that, especially for women, shattered Victorian bonds on sexuality and its expression. With his olive-tinted skin and his almond-shaped eyes, Valentino was the prototypical Latin lover, although in real life his romantic relationships tended toward the bizarre. A poor Italian immigrant, he followed a rags-to-riches trail to become a Hollywood superstar and three of his films are now regarded as classics of the silent screen. At the height of his career, he died of a perforated peptic ulcer, a condition that today can usually be prevented and, if not, can be treated effectively. His death unleashed a torrential public mourning that was as garish as it was pervasive. Moreover, the Valentino cult has persisted long after the names of other early film stars have been forgotten. To this day, more than a century after his birth, his devotees gather at his gravesite on the anniversary of his death.

Biography

Giovanni Guglielmi, a 36-year-old Italian veterinarian, and Gabriella Barbin, a refined and soft-spoken 33-year-old woman of French origins, married in 1889. Settling into middle class existence in Castellaneta, a town of 7000 just at the instep of the Italian boot, they had a daughter within a year, but she died shortly after her first birthday. Then came a son and then a second son, born on May 6, 1895, christened Rodolfo Piertro Filiberto Raffaele Guglielmi. The last of his given names was intended to honor the local nobleman who was presumably present at the christening. Two years later, a daughter completed the family. Young Rodolfo was close to his mother and sister, the beginning of a lifetime of easy attachments with women, and his sensitivity and fluency in French undoubtedly came from his mother. From early childhood, he had an exotic appearance, with terra cotta-colored skin and almond shaped eyes that suggested some Moorish or Byzantine ancestry. This visage may not have launched a thousand ships, as did Helen of Troy's, but it would become one of the most famous in the world.

The Guglielmi family moved to Taranto, a larger city on the coast of the Ionian Sea, when Rodolfo was nine. The new locale provided broader experiences and a more cosmopolitan perspective, but it brought tragedy when, a year later, Giovanni contracted malaria and died. His family was bereft, with each member grieving in different ways. For Rodolfo, there was a large component of guilt at failing to live up to his father's expectations. His school performance was poor and disobedience, lying, and contempt for authority became problematic. His late father's brothers and friends, feeling that Gabriella was too easily manipulated by her unruly child, convinced her to send him to a military school where discipline was strict, schoolwork rigorous, and living conditions monastic. However, the 12 year old did not give up his rebellious and lazy ways easily and he was nearly always in trouble for one reason or another. He did make somewhat of a mark in athletics where his natural abilities became evident. About the only lasting effect of military school was a cigarette habit he would retain for the rest of his life.

Leaving military school when faced with imminent expulsion, young Roldolfo was sent to an agricultural institute. His record was better there but when he came home after two years with a certificate of completion in hand, he reverted to his former indolent ways. He slept late after spending most nights in taverns and music halls, in the process becoming a very accomplished dancer, something that would stand him in good stead later. Tiring of provincial Taranto, he used his share of his father's inheritance to finance a trip to Paris where he was introduced to a level of sophistication undreamed of previously, including free and easy sex and a new dance from Argentina, the tango.

It was obvious to everyone, even to Rodolfo, that he was going nowhere. A new start in America seemed to offer a chance to get away from his record of failure. Thus, at the end of 1913, 18-year-old Rodolfo Guglielmi took ship from Naples, with a stop in Genoa, bound for New York. On the voyage, he spent most of his money to upgrade the second-class ticket his mother had purchased for him, worked at learning English, and danced and romanced several attractive female first-class passengers. By the time the ship docked in New York, his English was good enough to tell immigration authorities he was an "agriculturist" and that his middle name was "dei Marchesi," apparently in hopes people would assume he was descended from a marquis.

The young immigrant found housing with others recently arrived from Italy and turned to his immediate need for employment. He took a number of menial jobs but all were short-lived, for Rodolfo still had little taste for physical labor and even less for following any kind of directions. Just when failure seemed imminent, his talent and experience in social dancing came his rescue. He got a job at Maxim's Restaurant-Cabaret, a Manhattan watering hole where women—single or married, unescorted or with non-dancing escorts—came to dance during afternoons or evenings. Maxim's provided the male partners and very soon the most popular of them was "Signor Rodolfo." He was especially adept at the tango, a dance combining skillful steps and erotic steam. About this time came a name change, Guglielmo being difficult for the English speakers to pronounce, spell, or remember. Rodolfo claimed the middle name "di Valentina," implying a papal title conferred on an ancestor—although the name does not appear on either his birth or baptismal certificate—so he became "Rodolfo di Valentina." Later, in Hollywood, he would anglicize it to Rudolph Valentino.

One of several society women the taxi dancer came to know was Blanca de Saulles, a beautiful young Chilean trapped in an unhappy marriage to an older, wealthy American. Whether Rodolfo and Blanca had a sexual affair is uncertain but they certainly were close. When Blanca decided she wanted a divorce and needed help in proving her husband's infidelity, Rodolfo came forward and gave evidence naming one of his former dancing partners. In the summer of 1917, Blanca shot her husband during a dispute about custody of their child. It was a sensational, high society murder and the name of Rodolfo Guglielmi and the details of his testimony in the divorce hearing the previous year were in all the newspapers. Needing to get away from New York, he took a part in the road show cast of a musical production headed for California.

Rudy, as he had begun to style himself, left the theatrical company in San Francisco, once again finding himself a stranger looking for work in a strange city. He had a brief fling at vaudeville and even tried selling securities, but for his main employment he reverted to his earlier days as a gigolo, dancing for hire, before drifting southward to what seemed to be greener pastures in the burgeoning movie industry of Los Angeles. There he experienced some success, garnering small parts in various movies, but romantic or heroic roles did not seem to be in his future. The reason, quite simply, was a pervasive stereotyping in American culture of the early 20th century and in the film industry reflecting it: the heroes were square-jawed, broad-shouldered all-Americans like Douglas Fairbanks, whereas those with darker skins played heavies. Rudy's income increased progressively, although it remained far below the stratospheric levels of the superstars, as well as below his own standard of living.

Just when Rudy seemed stuck forever in secondary and stereotypic roles, his big break came. *The Four Horsemen of the Apocalypse* had become an international best seller as the first great novel to come out of World War I. It was an epic covering three generations, beginning in Argentina and ending on the battlefields of France, and the English translation had sold ten million copies in the United States alone. The studio owning the film rights assigned a woman named June Mathis to adopt the novel for the screen and also gave her a role in the casting. June Mathis had never met Rudolph Valentino (as he was now called) but she remembered seeing him in a minor movie role previously and she thought his exotic appearance and smoldering sex appeal were perfect for the lead role. The studio was reluctant but

June persisted, the first of several times she would prove critical in promoting Valentino's career. Although she was only eight years older than Rudy, their close relationship that developed over the years was like that of a mother and son.

Released at the end of 1920, *The Four Horsemen of the Apocalypse* was a smash hit, earning unanimous praise from critics and attracting huge crowds around the world. It also made its star a sensation. Not only had he delivered a riveting performance, but he also introduced a new type of acting, one in which the viewer had his (and especially her) emotions laid bare to their core.

Just before his career breakthrough, there had been a personal twist in Valentino's life that cannot be characterized as anything but bizarre. In September 1919 he met a rising young actress named Jean Acker and, seeing her several times, always in the company of others, over the next several weeks, he was quite taken with her. One day on a horseback ride, he asked her to marry him, an impulsive act and, just as impulsively, she accepted. The problem, which everyone except Valentino realized, was that Jean Acker was a lesbian and had many untidy emotional and sexual entanglements, always with other women. There was a wedding ceremony, after which Jean went to her hotel room and locked the door. Over the succeeding weeks and months, a steady stream of letter, telegrams, and telephone calls came from Rudy, imploring his bride to "come to your senses and give me an opportunity to prove my sincere love and eternal devotion to you." There were several physical confrontations that quickly became shouting and shoving matches. Finally, the true situation became clear to the unhappy bridegroom, as it had long been for everyone else, and he gave up. In January 1922, a little more than two years after their marriage ceremony and a few months after *The Four Horsemen of the Apocalypse* had made Valentino a movie star, they were divorced. He contended the marriage had not been consummated, and she did not dispute the claim.

Valentino's second big break came when he was cast in the lead role in *The Sheik*, playing an Arab chieftain who kidnaps and ravishes an English noblewoman. The leading lady succumbs joyously to the savagely virile, dark-skinned leading man and, at the film's release in October 1921, millions of women around the world would have given anything to trade places with her. If *The Four Horseman* made Valentino a star, *The Sheik* made him a superstar.

In the wake of his success, Rudy met the woman who would become his second wife. She went by the name of Natacha Rambova and in appearance she was every bit as exotic as her name. Actually, however, she was an American, born into affluence as Winifred Shaughnessy, who had spent her youth in boarding schools in England. She had taken the name Natacha Rambova during a love affair with a Russian ballet teacher. When she and Rudy met, she was past her dancing phase and worked as a designer of sets and costumes. There were some hints of lesbianism in her background, but she and Rudy fell in love.

Rudy and Natacha spent much of their spare time in Palm Springs and they headed there in May 1922, after completing filming of *Blood and Sand*, an important film in which Rudy played the leading role of a matador who dies in the bullring. Impulsively, the couple decided to get married. Rudy knew his divorce from Jean Acker would not be final for some months, but naïvely he reasoned that a marriage outside the country would present no legal problems. So the two of them, accompanied by a number of friends, drove across the border to Mexicali where they were married. Returning to Los Angeles, with an overnight stop in Palm Springs, they found themselves in the middle of a firestorm. A judge had given an informal opinion that the Mexicali marriage was invalid and the word "bigamist" was in every headline. Rudy was jailed for marrying while already wed and for "unlawful and felonious co-habiting." Advised by studio lawyers to get out of town, Natacha hurriedly took a train to her parents in upstate New York. Ultimately, after much legal maneuvering, the case was dismissed on grounds—proven in court by corroborating testimony but certainly untrue—that the couple had not spent the night together in Palm Springs after the wedding and, therefore, the marriage had not been consummated. Months later, on March 13, 1923, the final decree of Rudy's divorce from Jean Acker was entered in the Los Angeles County Superior Court and the next day he and Natacha were married by a Justice of the Peace in Crown Point, Indiana.

The Valentinos quickly settled into the life style of a Hollywood superstar couple. They bought a house in fashionable Whitley Heights, a forerunner of Beverly Hills, and set about furnishing it in staggeringly lavish ways. Each seemed to have endless supplies of fancy and opulent clothes and there was a fleet of expensive automobiles. They kept horses, which Rudy rode often, and a pair of enormous Dobermans that accompanied them everywhere. It was all was done with borrowed money, for Rudy's income, while substantial, was far below that of comparable movie stars and Natacha's financial contribution was modest. In July 1923, the pair took an extended trip to Europe where they toured all the areas frequented by the rich and famous and shopped incessantly. There was also a triumphal visit to Rudy's sister and brother in southern Italy.

There were more subtle changes in the actor for whom the movie magazine *Photoplay* coined the term "heart throb." He began to act more like the temperamental star, demanding control over scripts, feuding with directors, and fairly often stomping off the set when things did not please him. Many saw Natacha's influence in these personality changes and there is little doubt she goaded a husband she viewed as too passive. A dispute with the studio to which he was bound by contract simmered for some time, with Valentino feeling he was underpaid and that commitments to him had not been kept. There was protracted litigation, which finally ended with neither side winning and both saddled with extensive legal costs, something the Valentinos could ill-afford. Rudy then signed with another studio on rather more favorable terms with respect to autonomy and salary but with the important proviso that Natacha was excluded from any role in his making of pictures or any other aspect of his career.

By early 1923, when Rudy and Natacha had been wed for scarcely two years, the marriage began to show signs of deterioration. The new contract he signed was clearly a slap in her face, but there was probably a more fundamental problem: Rudy wanted children and Natacha did not. His provincial Italian background meant that children, especially a son and heir, were critically important and the wife's main role was to provide them. Natacha, by contrast had little interest in domestic activities or in catering to her husband's wants in any other way. Eventually, she took a lover, and then another, and then moved to New York, announcing that she and Rudy were taking a "marital vacation." At the end of 1925 they were divorced. He vowed never to wed again. Later, he did take up with Pola Negri, an exotic Polish actress then the rage in Hollywood, but there is no indication marriage was ever considered.

Rudolph Valentino played a starring role in 13 feature films between 1921 and 1926. Several of them—*The Four Horsemen of the Apocalypse, The Sheik,* and *Blood and Sand*—are regarded today as classics of the silent screen. Using sight but not sound, he was able to convey a range of emotions, most importantly that of a smoldering sexuality, arguably better than any actor before or since. The first talking picture would arrive only a few months after his death. How would Valentino have done in this new medium? One cannot be certain, but there is some basis for thinking he might have been in that small segment of silent performers who could make the transition to sound. He had a pleasant baritone voice and his accent was not pronounced. Of course, he would have had to learn a new style, one using more complex means of expressing emotion and one lacking in the exaggerated gestures and expressions characteristic of the silent era. But he possessed an abundance of natural ability, and he quite likely could have pulled it off.

Illness and death

Rudolph Valentino's image was that of a healthy, active, virile man, and this was one instance in which perception and reality corresponded closely. He had shown considerable athletic talent as a schoolboy in Italy, an interest he retained as an adult. Fencing, wrestling, and boxing were sports he engaged in regularly, and on one occasion he even sparred with Jack Dempsey, the heavyweight champion. He was always somewhat of a physical fitness nut and his exercise regimen was serialized in newspapers under the title "Valentino's Beauty Secrets." As soon as he could afford it, he kept a stable and went riding frequently; except when overruled by studio executives, he spurned the use of doubles for riding and similar activities in his movies.

He seemed to have been skeptical about doctors, perhaps reflecting a feeling common among the Italian peasantry during that era, and he tended to treat himself for occasional ailments such as respiratory infections. In fact, there is no record of him ever consulting a physician until his final illness. There must have been physical assessments periodically, for studios and their insurers required these before undertaking any major film, so presumably his state of good health was confirmed. Some of his associates recalled that, beginning in about 1922, he complained frequently of upset stomach and stomachaches. This was probably the onset of symptoms of peptic ulcer that would subsequently become so important. He also was a heavy smoker, although the adverse health effects of smoking were not really appreciated at the time.

In the summer of 1926, just after Natacha left him, he went on tour to promote his latest movie, *Son of Sheik*. A whirlwind of nonstop social activity proved ineffective in relieving his underlying unhappiness and sense of loss. Several associates remarked that he did not appear well and his butler later recalled him ingesting huge quantities of bicarbonate of soda. While in New York, on Saturday, August 14, he and a male friend went to a show and then dropped in on a party at a Park Avenue apartment. About 1:30 AM, Rudy complained of not feeling well and left the party, taking a taxi to his hotel. When daylight dawned, friends found him violently ill, with excruciating abdominal pain, and they sent for a doctor. The doctor's examination revealed a rigid abdomen and a rapid pulse, suggesting some intra-abdominal catastrophe. An ambulance took him to the Polyclinic Hospital, arriving about noon. There may have some delay, this being Saturday, but at 4:30 pm Dr. Harold Meeker began an abdominal operation. The hospital reported the diagnosis as perforated gastric ulcer and acute appendicitis. Later, Meeker would state "there was a hole in the stomach the size of a dime."

The morning after surgery, Sunday, Valentino awakened and made jokes with those at his bedside. His temperature was elevated and the hospital reports seemed guarded but Rudy himself minimized his condition as being "just a little indisposed and I will soon be all right." Meanwhile, the three women in his life vied for the inside position as the deeply concerned, loving mate. Jean Acker, partner in his first marriage which all agreed was unconsummated, announced she had canceled a planned trip to Europe and would remain close to Rudy in his hour of need. Natacha Rambova, second wife and the one he had not gotten over, cabled from France that she was "praying hourly for your recovery" and hinted at reconciliation. Pola Negri, the current love interest, told the Hollywood press that she wanted desperately to rush to his bedside but was in the middle of filming and the studio would not hear of it.

Bulletins issued daily by his physicians gave his temperature, pulse rate, and respiratory rate. On Tuesday and Wednesday, his temperature was 103 degrees, but by Thursday it had fallen to 101 and the following day was normal. The doctors announced that the crisis had passed and no more daily bulletins would be issued. The patient began taking soup and Vichy water orally. He ordered roses for his nurse and asked if he might continue his recuperation at his hotel.

However, later on Friday, August 20, came an alarming turn for the worse. He complained of severe pain on the left side of his chest and abdomen and his temperature rose again, to 103. Consultants were called in and it soon became clear that the actor was critically ill. His condition deteriorated and on Sunday evening his agent sent for a priest. Rudy had long since lapsed as a Roman Catholic, twice married outside the church and twice divorced. He was only intermittently awake, but the priest reported hearing his confession and granting absolution, and then the cleric administered the last rites of the Roman church. The following morning, Valentino slipped into a coma and later, at 12:10 pm, Monday, August 23, 1926, the 31-year-old actor— arguably the best-known male film personality in the world—died, alone except for three doctors and two nurses.

The death certificate, prepared hastily by the chief resident physician, Dr. William B. Rawls, contained many errors. Valentino's real surname was misspelled, his father's first name and his mother's country of birth were both erroneous, and the deceased's place of residence was given as the Ambassador Hotel. In a press conference, Dr. Rawls told the press he could not be certain about the cause of death since no autopsy was done, but the clinical diagnosis was "ruptured gastric ulcer with general peritonitis . . . septic pneumonia and septic endocarditis." What seemed to be a hint of uncertainty about his illness and why he died would prove to be fodder for generations of conspiracy theorists.

News of Valentino's death brought an outpouring of shock and grief on a scale not seen before, at least in America, and probably not since. His two ex-wives and the actress who was his current love interest (and, according to her, his one true love) tried to outdo each other in their grieving. Tributes came from every corner of the entertainment world, including such luminaries as Charlie Chaplin and Gloria Swanson. Major newspapers devoted extensive coverage to everything remotely connected with the actor and tried in their editorial columns to assess his place in history. At least two women fans, one in New York and the other in London, committed suicide surrounded by pictures of Valentino, apparently feeling that life without him was not worth living. There was a large element of disbelief in the response of the general public: how could this handsome and athletic young man, the very embodiment of vitality and physical perfection, be struck down so suddenly?

Valentino's body was moved from the hospital to a funeral chapel a few blocks away, where it was embalmed and placed in an elaborate and expensive casket for public viewing. By dawn the day after he died, a crowd eventually estimated at thirty thousand began filling the streets around the funeral parlor and, when a heavy rainstorm began, a riot erupted. The unruly crowd surged against a large plate glass window, shattering it and sending more than a hundred to hospitals. Later in the afternoon, the doors were opened to the public and by the time they were closed at midnight some fifty thousand people had passed by the bier. Police characterized it as the most frenzied and disorderly crowd they had ever seen in New York. The funeral parlor was stripped bare of furnishings and floral displays and only a phalanx of policemen prevented souvenir hunters from attacking the casket and body. The next day, Wednesday the 25th, was only slightly more orderly, as some twenty to forty thousand filed past the bier. Then the people in charge decided things had gone far enough, and they announced that henceforth only friends and associates would admitted to view the body.

New York law required the funeral to be held within seven days of death, and it took place on the last possible day, Monday, August 30. The setting was St. Malachy's Catholic Church, with High Requiem Mass celebrated by Father Edward F. Leonard, the priest who had administered last rites to the dying Valentino. Admission was by printed and numbered invitation only and the mourners represented a who's who of the New York entertainment industry. Opera singers sang Gounod's *Ave Maria* and Massenet's *Elegy* and the organist played Chopin's *Funeral March*. The crowd was orderly compared to the public display at the funeral home several days earlier, although there was much weeping and a few attendees who seemed to lapse into unconsciousness. When it was over, the casket was returned to the funeral parlor to await its final trip to California. The funeral train, consisting of a baggage car containing the silver-bronze casket and a special coach for the official party, left Grand Central Station on the evening of September 2. It was hitched to the Lake Shore Limited and then in Chicago to the Golden State Limited. All along the way, crowds gathered in mostly-silent tribute, drawing comparisons with Abraham Lincoln's funeral train.

The second funeral service took place on Tuesday, September 7, at the Beverly Hills Church of the Good Shepherd, with Father Michael J. Mullins celebrating High Mass. It was similar to the New York service and the audience included all the Hollywood luminaries. The California funeral had been planned just as meticulously as the New York version, although somewhat curiously the issue of burial had received scant attention. June Mathis, Valentino's mentor, came forward at the last minute with what she presented as a temporary solution, while plans for an elaborate memorial (consisting of statues of Valentino in his most famous roles), and more importantly for its financing, could be worked out. Mathis had purchased crypts in the mausoleum of Hollywood Memorial Cemetery at her mother's death several years earlier and there were niches intended for Mathis and her husband. She suggested Valentino occupy one of the as-yet open places temporarily. Thus, after the Beverly Hills funeral and a last trip of the cortege along Santa Monica Boulevard, Rudolph Valentino came to rest in what was viewed as temporary quarters. But June Mathis died of a heart attack less than a year after her protégé and was interred next to him, and her husband returned to his native Italy where he lost interest in being buried next to his wife. Valentino's executors eventually paid him for the niche the actor occupied and it became his final and permanent resting place.

But it was not quite over. The mausoleum in Hollywood Memorial Cemetery (later renamed Hollywood Forever) quickly became, and has remained, a site of pilgrimage. Fans of the actor, many of them wearing sheik costumes or heavy black veils, regularly gather on August 23 at 12:10 PM, the day and hour of his death in New York, apparently unaware of the three hour difference between Eastern and Pacific time zones. Readings and eulogies are given; for many years the speakers were people who knew Valentino but now the mourners are all born after the actor's death.

Probably the best known of the Valentino mourners was the "Lady in Black," who appeared each year, beginning shortly after his death and continuing for many years, and deposited a single red rose at the tomb. Many claimed to be this person, but her identity was ultimately established as a

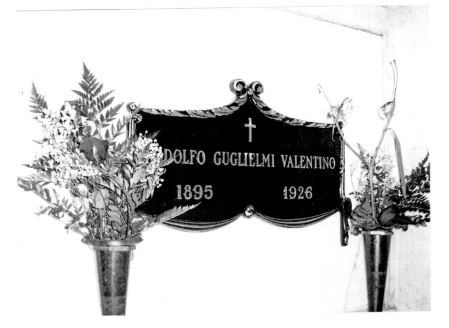

Figure 7.2 Valentino tomb, Hollywood Forever

former vaudeville dancer and violinist with the stage name of Ditra Flambé. She claimed that Valentino had visited her once when she was ill and urged her to carry on this ritual after his death, but there is little objective evidence the two ever met. During Valentino's lifetime, and especially in the wake of his death, more than a few women claimed the actor fathered their children. Cemetery caretakers reported that, for years after his death, pregnant women would visit the tomb, announcing they had been impregnated by him.

Immortality comes in different ways and in Rudolph Valentino's case there is at least one more manifestation: it is his silhouette, in one of his most famous roles, that for many years adorned packages of Sheik® condoms.

Medical Perspectives

The Polyclinic Hospital released a public statement shortly after Valentino's surgery that the actor had "a perforated gastric ulcer and acute appendicitis" and these diagnoses seem to have been accepted without question by subsequent biographers. However, the simultaneous existence of these two conditions would be purely coincidental and therefore highly improbable. It is much more likely that the perforated gastric ulcer and its spillage of stomach contents (acid and bacteria) caused generalized inflammation of the membrane lining the abdominal cavity and its organs, including the appendix. Thus, while inflammation of the appendix would be seen both grossly and microscopically, it was almost certainly secondary to the perforated ulcer and not a primary event, as it would be with acute appendicitis. Even in the highly unlikely event the two conditions did happen to exist at the same time in the same person, the perforated ulcer would pose the more immediate and serious threat to life.

Peptic (a term meaning related to digestion) ulcers are divided into gastric and duodenal types, depending on whether they are located in the stomach or duodenum, the first portion of the small intestine adjacent to the stomach. Regardless of location, however, all peptic ulcers arise from the same mechanism and cause the same signs and symptoms. Cells in the stomach wall normally secrete acid, which is important in the digestive process, and the traditional concept is that excessive acid secretion literally erodes or eats away the surface of the stomach or duodenum, forming the ulcer. As will be explained later, recent research has cast doubt on acidity as the primary or sole feature, although stomach acid unquestionably plays an important role in the disease.

Peptic ulcer is common. It is estimated that 10% of people have one at some time in their lives. The condition has traditionally been considered a disease of modern civilization with its high stress, a relationship based on the known tendency for acid secretion to increase with anxiety and emotional tension. Acid secretion is also stimulated by certain highly seasoned foods and alcohol, as well as by smoking. Thus, the classic ulcer candidate is the person, often a male in a high stress job such as an executive position, who smokes cigarettes, drinks excessively, and eats erratically. The cardinal symptom of peptic ulcer is upper abdominal pain, which may be described as burning or gnawing or boring, typically when the stomach is empty, and alleviated by ingesting antacids or bland foods such as milk. The diagnosis can be suspected on clinical grounds but usually requires confirmation by gastrointestinal x-rays (involving drinking a barium solution which is impervious to x-rays and therefore outlines the shallow depression of the ulcer) or direct visualization with an endoscope passed through the mouth and into the stomach.

Peptic ulcer is a chronic condition but it can in some instances lead to acute and serious complications. If the ulcer extending into the wall of the stomach or duodenum should happen to erode into a blood vessel, there will be bleeding and sometimes it can be massive. Such bleeding becomes evident by the affected individual vomiting blood or passing large quantities of tar-like material (representing blood modified by passage through the small and large intestines) rectally. Acute and severe hemorrhage of this type can be life threatening and usually requires emergency abdominal surgery to control it. Another and even more ominous complication is perforation, where the ulcer erodes through the full thickness of the stomach or duodenum. This causes excruciatingly severe pain and a rigid, board-like abdomen because the stomach contents spill into the abdominal cavity and set up inflammation of the lining membranes. Immediate surgery to close the perforation and usually to remove the diseased area of the ulcer is essential. Even with prompt operation, however, the complication was often fatal until antibiotics became available in the middle of the 20th century. Nowadays, giving powerful antibiotic drugs along with prompt surgery usually leads to recovery.

The mainstay of medical treatment of peptic ulcer has long been antacids, agents that neutralize acidity. Originally, sodium bicarbonate was used but, since sodium is readily absorbed, continued heavy use can cause complications from excessive sodium load. Salts of calcium, magnesium, and aluminum are absorbed to much lesser degrees and are therefore preferable. The two most widely used antacid tablets, Tums® and Rolaids®, both consist mainly of calcium carbonate. Antacids of this type come as tablets or liquid but in all cases they act by neutralizing stomach acid already present. A major advance was the development in the 1970s of drugs that suppress the production and/or release of acid, known as H2 blockers and proton pump inhibitors. H2 blockers, the first to become available, act by blocking the action of histamine, a stimulant of acid secretion, and proton pump inhibitors suppress the mechanism that pumps acid into the stomach from acid-making cells. Since the action of these newer drugs is to inhibit acid release, rather than to neutralize it, there is a delay of 30-60 minutes between ingesting the drug and seeing an effect. Originally, they required a physician's prescription but in recent years low doses of H2 blocker were made available over the counter.

The long and deeply held concept of the primary role of stomach acid in causing peptic ulcer was revolutionized by the 1982 discovery of a specific bacterial organism that seemed to be responsible. Two Australian investigators, J. Robin Warren and Barry J. Marshall, received the 2005 Nobel Prize in Medicine or Physiology for identifying a spiral-shaped microorganism that weakens the protective mucous coating of the stomach and adjacent small intestine, allowing acid to get through to the sensitive lining beneath. This erodes the surface, forming an ulcer or sore. Known as *Helicobacter pylori (H. pylori)*, the bacterium represents the primary factor in at least 90% of peptic ulcers and, while acid is involved, its role is secondary.

The means by which H. pylori is transmitted is not known with certainty but ingestion of contaminated food or water seems most likely. Of several methods to diagnose *H. pylori* infection, the one used most commonly is a blood test for antibodies against the organism. The discovery of this organism revolutionized the concepts of how peptic ulcers develop and how they should be treated. Antacids and drugs to inhibit acid secretion remain important components of therapy but the critical treatment is an appropriate antibiotic. The regimen used most commonly, known as triple therapy, includes two antibiotics (such as metronidazole, tetracycline, or amoxicillin) and either an acid suppressor or an agent to protect the stomach lining (such as bismuth subsalicylate or Pepto-Bismol®) given for two weeks. The response rate to this kind of regimen is quite good.

Surgery has a limited but definite place in the modern management of peptic ulcer. As noted previously, it can be life saving as an emergency procedure if there is either extensive hemorrhage or perforation. Several different operations were developed during the late 18th and early 19th centuries to treat ulcers that failed to respond to medical therapy. These operations, mostly based on the now-discredited theory of acid's primary role, involved different approaches to decreasing acid production such as removing a substantial portion of the stomach or cutting the nerves to the stomach. They have been largely, if not quite entirely, obviated by newer medical approaches.

What would have been Rudolph Valentino's fate if his medical problem had occurred 75 years after it actually did? His history of abdominal complaints and frequent antacid ingestion would have prompted an investigation including an upper gastrointestinal x-ray study and/or endoscopy of the stomach and either of these studies would establish the diagnosis of gastric ulcer. If blood, breath, or stool tests indicated *H. pylori* infection, therapy with one or two antibiotics and an acid reducer or a protector of the stomach lining would probably cure the problem. Had he suffered perforation of the stomach, as he actually did, emergency surgery to repair the perforation would be necessary but, with powerful modern antibiotics, the attendant infection could almost surely be overcome. Thus, modern treatment would almost certainly have led to Rudolph Valentino's survival.

SOURCES

Leider, Emily W. *Dark Lover*. Farrar, Strauss and Giroux. New York. 2003

Bothan Neil. *Valentino: The First Superstar*. Metro Publishing Ltd. London. 2002

www.cdc.gov/ulcer/md.htm. Accessed January 25, 2005.

http://digestive.niddk.nih.gov/ddiseases/pubs/hpylori. Accessed January 25, 2005

CHAPTER 8

LOU GEHRIG AND
AMYOTROPHIC LATERAL SCLEROSIS

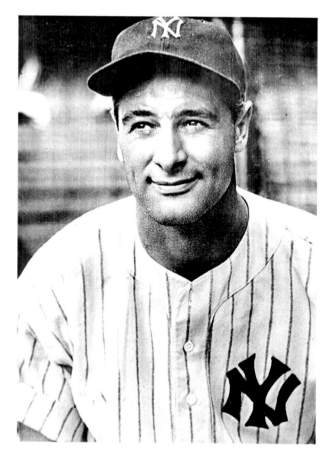

Figure 8.1 Lou Gehrig: Pride of the Yankees
(National Baseball Hall of Fame, Cooperstown, NY)

Baseball, known as "the great American pastime," is really more an American institution, and for some an obsession. Its best practitioners become national heroes, enshrined in an elaborate Hall of Fame and remembered and revered long after their playing days end. No resident of baseball's pantheon occupies a more honored position than does Lou Gehrig, first baseman for the New York Yankees in the 1920s and 1930s. He was, of course, a marvelous athlete and he established many records, including an especially notable one for endurance. But he was more than an athlete, more than someone who simply possessed extraordinary physical abilities. Quiet, modest, and self-effacing, Gehrig had the kind of personal qualities and character every parent desires in a son. Then, at the height of his career, he developed a rare neurologic disease—one with which name will forever be linked—that ended his playing days and within two years caused his death. In one of fate's supreme ironies, a man whose neuromuscular coordination was virtually superhuman fell victim to a disease that destroys the nervous system's ability to control muscular function. Much has been learned about "Lou Gehrig's disease" since he died of it nearly 70 years ago, but its outcome has changed little.

Biography

Among the millions of immigrants flooding America's shores during the decade or two before 1900—the "wretched refuse" of the Lazarus poem—two who came from Germany were Heinrich Gehrig in 1888 and Christina Fack in 1899. They met in New York shortly after Christina's arrival and were married the following year, settling with other German immigrants in the Yorkville section of Manhattan. Heinrich's trade was artistic metalworking, a craft that paid reasonably well but was not often in demand. Therefore, Christina needed to work—doing housework for others, taking in laundry, and using her considerable cooking skills. Even so, the Gehrig family faced poverty more or less continuously and their life was anything but easy in other ways, not least because of the anti-German prejudice around the time of World War I.

Heinrich and Christina had four children but only the second, a boy born in 1903, survived past early childhood. Given the name Heinrich Ludwig, quickly anglicized to Henry Louis, he soon came to be called Lou. Christina was a domineering woman and Heinrich seemed to stay in the background much of the time. Young Lou grew up essentially as an only child and, as soon as he was able, he helped his mother in her domestic work. Leisure time was scarce, but he was able to play various street games occasionally and very early he demonstrated an aptitude for sports. Formal education for boys of Lou's status typically did not extend beyond grammar school, but

Christina was adamant about her son getting more and, as usual, she prevailed. Lou gained entrance into Manhattan's High School of Commerce, an institution known for the value of its training in bookkeeping, typing, clerical work, and other commercial skills.

At Commerce, the strapping young man was introduced to organized athletics and his abilities in soccer, football, and especially baseball soon became obvious. He still helped his mother by delivering cooking and laundry and he took various odd jobs after school and on weekends. These activities cut into time for practice but he nevertheless became a star in several sports. The Commerce High baseball team was especially successful in his last year and a game with Lane Tech, the high school champion team of Chicago, was arranged. Christina Gehrig considered sports as a waste of time and to get her permission to make the trip to Chicago required several hours of pleading from Lou. Ultimately, she consented, albeit grudgingly. The game received considerable coverage in the newspapers and ten thousand people gathered in Wrigley Field to see the playoff between the high school champions of the two largest cities. Commerce, behind by 8-6 in the ninth inning, loaded the bases when Lou came to bat. He hit the ball clear out of the park—a home run of true major league dimensions—to win the game for Commerce.

The Chicago game brought considerable fame to the Commerce High team and to its slugger, and it raised the possibility of Lou playing baseball professionally. But Mom Gehrig would have none of it. To her, baseball was "a bunch of nonsense" and "a game for bummers" and her son was to continue his education. Columbia University, where Mom had recently landed a job as cook in the Sigma Nu fraternity house, expressed an interest in the young athlete and offered a football scholarship. Lou was only an average student and it took several months of diligent study for him to meet the entrance requirements, but in the fall of 1921 he matriculated at Columbia in the engineering program. Money remained a problem and Lou needed a job waiting tables at a fraternity and a variety of odd jobs to be able to stay in school. He was a solid performer in football, playing in both the line and the backfield, but it was in baseball that he starred. He pitched and played first base and outfield, and his gargantuan home runs were long remembered by those who saw them. In the spring of his sophomore year, a scout for the New York Yankees saw him hit one estimated to travel 450 feet, so impressive that the Yankee management made an attractive offer: 1500 dollars to sign a contract and 2000 dollars for the remainder of the 1923 season. Mom Gehrig remained skeptical but the money represented a veritable fortune, so she eventually relented.

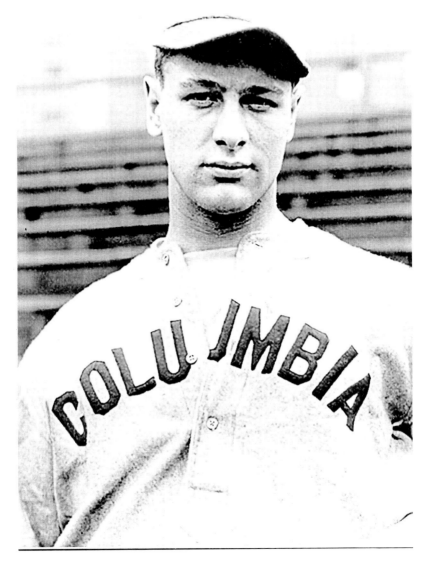

Figure 8.2 Lou Gehrig at Columbia University

When he reported to the New York Yankees in June 1923, no one questioned Lou's hitting ability but he was far from a polished baseball player and his fielding skills were particularly problematic. As a big, muscular left hander, both batting and throwing, his natural position was first base but he was inconsistent in fielding ground balls and digging errant throws out of the dirt. After a few weeks on the Yankee bench, he was sent to the farm team in Hartford, Connecticut for "seasoning." He started slowly at Hartford but then picked up and ended the season with a respectable .304

115

batting average, including many extra base hits. He came back to the Yankees for the last several weeks of the major league season and played in a few games. The next spring found him with the Yankees for spring training, where he improved his fielding with the help of the talented first baseman, Wally Pipp. However, Gehrig still seemed a little raw for the big leagues and, moreover, the Yankees were covered at first base, so he was sent back to Hartford for the rest of the 1924 season. He had a fantastic year there: 134 games with 37 home runs and a batting average of .383, albeit with 23 fielding errors. Called up to the Yankees at season's end, Lou played in ten games and had six hits in 12 at-bats.

During spring training in 1925, Gehrig seemed destined to again understudy Pipp, who had turned in his best performance the preceding year. However, Lou was not sent down to the minors. On June 1, he got into a game as a pinch hitter. Though no one could know it at the time, it was a day to be remembered, for it was the beginning of a record that would stand as one of the most remarkable in the history of baseball. The following day, Wally Pipp was hit in the head during batting practice, so Gehrig filled in for him. The next day, the manager told Lou, "You're my first baseman today. Today and from now on." It would be 2,130 games and nearly 14 years before the Yankees would play a game without Lou Gehrig, a record considered as one of the two or three most hallowed of a game that more than any other rests on statistics and records. The streak was widely regarded as one that would never be matched, although many years later it would be.

The Yankee team on which Gehrig became a regular would soon become legendary but in his first year, 1925, there was little indication of what was coming. Key personnel had injuries and illnesses and dissension flared from time to time, with the result that the Yankees finished the season in seventh place. Gehrig had a good season for a rookie, with 20 home runs and a batting average of .295, and he worked conscientiously to improve his fielding. The next year, things began to jell for the Yankees and they won the American League pennant, with Lou hitting .313 and driving in 135 runs. Although the New York team lost to the St. Louis Cardinals in the 1926 World Series, they would prove the next year that they were the best in baseball at the time, and many today consider the 1927 Yankees the best team ever. The leader was the indomitable Babe Ruth, regarded by many as the best to ever play the game, and he and Gehrig formed the heart of a batting order that became known as "Murderers' Row."

Much has been made of interpersonal tensions between Ruth and Gehrig. It is difficult to imagine two more different personalities. The flamboyant Ruth was a Rabelaisian character who overindulged in nearly everything: eating, drinking, womanizing, and gambling. No form of debauchery seemed beyond him. He could be loud, boisterous, crude, and boorish, but he represented good "copy" to the news media and as a result his public image was that of a warm, generous, and charming boy who happened to occupy the body of a superb athlete. Gehrig, on the other hand, was unassuming and anything but colorful, and therefore uninteresting to reporters. He held baseball in deep reverence and respected authority, continuing to live with his parents even after he became an established star. He enjoyed a substantial income (although not nearly as high as Ruth). His top salary was $39,000 in 1938, equivalent to over a half-million in 2007 dollars, but nameless utility infielders receive that much today.

Different as they were in almost everything, there was one way in which Gehrig and Ruth complimented each other perfectly: hitting the baseball. Nowhere was this more evident than during 1927, a season in which the Yankees won the American League pennant by 19 games and then proceeded to demolish the Pittsburgh Pirates in four straight games of the World Series. Babe and Lou batted third and fourth, respectively, in the order and for most of the season were in a seesaw contest to see who could hit the most home runs. Toward the end, Ruth forged ahead, ending the regular season with 60, a record considered unbreakable for many years. Gehrig hit 47 home runs for the year, batted .373, and drove in a record 175 runs. The last statistic is all the more remarkable in view of the fact that, following Ruth in the batting order, Gehrig batted with the bases empty at least 60 times. Although it was only his second full year in the majors, he was voted the league's Most Valuable Player. The Yankees won the pennant and the World Series again in 1928, although not quite as convincingly as the year before, and Gehrig's home run total fell off to 27 but he again led the league in runs batted in, with 142.

It looked as though the Yankees would go on forever, but in 1929 their fortunes sank along with the stock market. The final blow came late in the season when Miller Huggins, the diminutive manager who had been a father figure to Lou Gehrig, died of an infection. The Yankees seemed to be in decline for the next three years, but they came roaring back to win the pennant and the World Series in 1932. By this time, however, Babe Ruth was nearing 40 and his lifelong dissipations began to catch up with him. He would hang on until he was finally traded in 1934, but his last several years were mostly downhill. Meanwhile, the younger and seemingly indestructible Gehrig continued to turn in stellar performances. Over the nine years from 1929 through 1937, his batting average ranged from .329 to .379, his home run totals from 32 to 49, and his runs batted in from 119 to 184, the latter an American League record that stands to this day. He was voted Most

Valuable Player in the American League in 1927 and again in 1936 and in 1934 he led the league in batting average, home runs, and runs batted in, giving him baseball's most coveted batting distinction, the Triple Crown, won only nine times during the hundred-plus years of the league.

While the handsome athlete was becoming one of America's greatest celebrities, his personal life continued, at least in the eyes of many, to be deadly dull and ordinary. He lived at home with his parents, dated infrequently, and stayed out of the spotlight, except of course on the baseball field. All this changed one evening in 1932 season when the Yankees were in Chicago to play the White Sox. Lou and a few other players were invited to a small party, the kind of invitation he usually declined. This time, however, he accepted, probably with the intent of making an appearance and then going to bed early. Also at the party was Eleanor Twitchell, an attractive 25-year-old woman who dressed and acted the part of a "twenties flapper." Eleanor and Lou could hardly have been more different—she the vivacious party girl and he the strong but very silent athlete—but it was for both love at first sight (well, technically not first sight, for they had been introduced once at the ball park in 1928, but neither had any clear recollection of it). Their courtship proceeded at what Eleanor and most others considered a glacial pace. Lou telephoned frequently, sometimes daily while he was on road trips, and whenever he was in Chicago they would have lunch or dinner, or both, together. Finally, Lou proposed marriage, although Eleanor had undoubtedly arranged and orchestrated the proposal.

It was abundantly clear to Eleanor that Christina Gehrig represented a major problem. She had not approved of any of Lou's previous girl friends and now that there was a serious one, there was no chance the relationship would find favor with her. Eleanor tried, inviting Mom Gehrig for a visit to Chicago, but it was hopeless. Lou attempted for a time to remain the loving and obedient son he had always been, but ultimately he did something he had scarcely ever done before: he issued an edict: "Eleanor will come first." The couple found an apartment and a small wedding was planned for September 29, 1933. Mom Gehrig announced that she would not attend because, she said, she might create a scene, so Lou took matters into his own hands. When he got home from the ballpark on September 28, he called the mayor of the suburb to come over to their apartment and marry them, with cleaners and painters as witnesses.

Eleanor and Lou lived one of sport's greatest romances as their love flourished and blossomed. Eleanor introduced Lou to several cultural activities. He was fascinated with ballet, marveling at the athleticism involved, and he became a rather serious opera lover. He was especially taken with Wagnerian operas, where his childhood fluency in German helped, and his favorite was *Tristan und Isolde*. She, in turn, became a dedicated and knowledgeable baseball fan. Relationships between the two Mrs. Gehrigs remained problematic, but eventually came somewhat of an armed truce.

Baseball, far more than any other sport, has always been obsessed with records and statistics. Because the game has changed so little over more than a century, comparisons have much more meaning than is the case with other sports. Lou Gehrig's career—13 full seasons and small parts of two others—was shorter than many other great players, and his lifetime statistics need to be interpreted in that light. For example, Ty Cobb played 24 years, Willie Mays and Henry Aaron each 23, and Babe Ruth 22. Nevertheless, Gehrig's record of 23 "grand slam" home runs (i.e., home runs with the bases full) stands at the top of all major leaguers and he ranks fourth on the all-time list for runs batted in, with 1995 during his career. But, of course, the record for which he is most remembered that of playing in 2,130 consecutive regular season games (if exhibition and World Series games were included, there would be many more). The streak began, as noted previously, in early 1924 and it lasted 14 years. No one really seemed aware of it until, midway through the 1933 season, when a sportswriter, apparently with time on his hands, discovered that Gehrig would soon break the existing record. As he did break it and then as he continued to set a new record every time he played, there was speculation as to the reason for his endurance. Baseball has an adage that one can play only as long as the legs last, and Lou had powerful legs, legs that carried his large body at an amazing speed. Some postulated an emotional cause, an obsessive nature that helped him play through the inevitable injuries. Two physicians from Columbia University assessed his cardiovascular records and pointed to his slow pulse and normal blood pressure. Lou himself would casually dismiss theories involving unusual devotion to duty, saying he simply wanted to play baseball; if pressed, he would suggest his low-key and relatively abstemious lifestyle might be responsible.

Gehrig's consecutive game streak was considered unassailable. Night games and long travel times; the increasing length and intensity of major league baseball; and an inexorable inflation in size, speed, and athletic ability all seemed to indicate that no single player could play in every single game over 14 seasons—or so it was reasoned. But there is an old sports adage that records are made to be broken, and indeed this "unbreakable" mark ultimately fell. It was broken by Cal Ripken, Jr., another "nice guy" who quietly came to work and did his job every day over 2,632 games from 1982 to 1998. On the day in 1995 he broke Gehrig's record, Ripken's team established the Cal Ripken/Lou Gehrig Fund for Neuromuscular Research, funded with all the money from ticket sales to that game. It was something

Gehrig would have liked. When Ripken was inducted into baseball's Hall of Fame in 2007, his acceptance speech drew heavily on his deep respect for the hero whose record he had bettered.

<u>Illness and Death</u>

In 1938 Gehrig was in his 36th year, somewhat past the prime for a high intensity sport like baseball but an age where many players are still able to perform in a perfectly acceptable manner. The year turned out to be disappointing, with his .295 batting average and 114 runs batted in his lowest in these categories since 1925 and 1926, respectively, but nevertheless better than most other major leaguers. Moreover, the Yankees won the pennant easily and demolished the Chicago Cubs in the World Series, and Lou and everyone else assumed 1938 was just a bit of an off year. He had seen players hang on too long and resolved that this would not happen with him, so he and Eleanor decided tentatively that the 1939 season be his last.

Spring training in 1939 brought concerns that could not be ignored. Gehrig had obvious problems with both hitting and fielding and even seemed to stumble and almost fall a few times in the clubhouse. His response was to take more batting and fielding practice in the belief that he could work it out. Several sportswriters asked if the time had not come to end the consecutive game streak, but the Yankee manager made it clear that Lou himself would make any such decision. The Yankees opened the season on April 20 and in eight games over the next 13 days Gehrig managed only four hits, all singles, and he made two errors. He told the manager the time had come for him to stand aside and on May 2, 1939 in Detroit, the Yankees played their first game in nearly 14 years without Lou Gehrig in the lineup.

Over the next few weeks, Gehrig struggled into his uniform before each game and sat on the bench. As team captain, a title he had held since 1935, he walked to home plate to turn in the batting order to the umpires before each game, but all could see his condition deteriorating rapidly. In early June he and Eleanor traveled to Rochester, Minnesota, for an evaluation at the Mayo Clinic. Tests over several days led to a diagnosis of amyotrophic lateral sclerosis (ALS), a disease of the spinal cord in which the tracts that carry impulses between brain and muscles deteriorate. The Mayo Clinic issued a statement giving the diagnosis and indicating that Lou's playing days were over (but stating that he could serve "in some executive capacity"). Eleanor was told the course would be progressive and ultimately fatal, but she directed that this information be kept from Lou. He participated in two different trials of experimental treatment, the first involving histamine under the direction of the Mayo Clinic and the second testing high-dose vitamin E injections under a New York City physician. Both researchers were very optimistic about their treatments, and Gehrig seemed to share their enthusiasm, but it turned out that neither had any influence on the course of the disease, in Gehrig or anyone else. Whether or not Lou guessed the prognosis as his condition deteriorated is uncertain.

New information about Gehrig's final months has come to light very recently, with the discovery of his extended correspondence with Dr. Paul O'Leary of the Mayo Clinic. The two had met during Lou's initial visit to Rochester and they forged a close friendship. O'Leary was a dermatologist and his involvement in Gehrig's care was indirect, so the tone of the correspondence is mainly that of friendship, albeit with some aspect of a doctor-patient relationship. Gehrig's letters, written in his own firm, masculine hand, describe his gradual deterioration in physical function and his hopes that things will get better. O'Leary's typewritten replies are encouraging and supportive, although at times blatantly wrong, such as his suggestion of a 45% chance of recovery. O'Leary was more honest in letters to Eleanor, finally telling her what she already knew, that Mayo Clinic patients with this disease "have not done well." Perhaps Lou guessed as much toward the end, for in one of his last letters he wrote "I don't mean to be pessimistic, but one cannot help wonder how far this thing will go."

Following Lou's return from the Mayo Clinic, the Yankee organization hurriedly made plans for a "Gehrig Appreciation Day" on July 4, 1939. It turned out to be one of the most memorable events in sports history. All the old teammates, including Babe Ruth, were there and there were gifts and speeches. But the more than 62,000 fans in attendance wanted to hear from the honoree and, when it was first announced that he was "too moved to speak," they would have none of it, shouting his name in unison. And so, in perhaps the most poignant moment ever in sports, Gehrig walked unsteadily to the microphone and pulled a piece of paper from his pocket. It was a short but moving speech, one he had written the night before. Particularly memorable were his opening sentences: "Fans, for the past two weeks you have been reading about a bad break I got. Yet today I consider myself the luckiest man on the face of the earth." It was mostly captured on film and Gehrig's poignant words are still remembered today, generations later.

Baseball had other recognitions to confer. In December 1939 the Baseball Writers Association voted Gehrig into the National Baseball Hall of Fame in a special election. At the same time, the New York Yankees announced that uniform number 4 was being retired and would never be worn by a Yankee again, the first time this had ever been done by a major league baseball team.

The popular mayor of New York, Fiorello La Guardia, invited Gehrig to serve as a parole commissioner, believing he would be a role model for young people in trouble. After careful consideration and with Eleanor's strong encouragement, Lou accepted the offer. The job involved making decisions about the time of release for prisoners given indefinite sentences and it was anything but an honorary position. Lou threw himself into it with the same commitment he had given to baseball, spending long hours studying personnel records of street criminals, hoodlums, prostitutes, con artists and others he had previously had little to do with. Nearly every day, Eleanor drove him from home to his office in lower Manhattan. Some days he went to prison facilities at Rikers Island or the Tombs. Appointed to a ten-year term on January 2, 1940, he actually served only a little more than a year before his condition had deteriorated to a point he could no longer function.

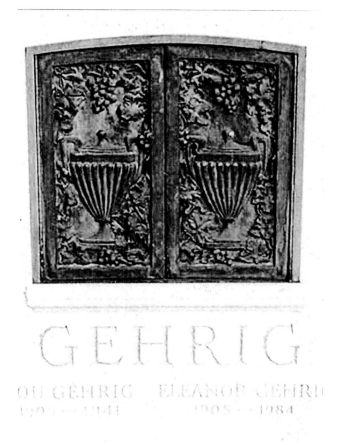

Figure 8.4 Gehrig tombstone (with erroneous birth year),
Kensico Cemetery, Valhalla, NY (Courtesy of Randy McCoy)

Lou spent his last few months at home, with Eleanor his constant companion and caregiver. There were a number of visits by friends and former teammates and an occasional outing to Yankee Stadium. But the downhill course was inexorable and eventually he had lost every activity he cherished. The legs that had made him a surprisingly fast base runner and the arms that had propelled many baseballs out of the park were useless. He died in his sleep, with Eleanor at his bedside, on June 2, 1941, 17 days before his 38th birthday. There was a public viewing at a church on 76th Street and Central Park West, with thousands filing past his bier. After a very brief funeral service at the Christ Protestant Episcopal Church in Riverdale, the body was cremated and the ashes interred in Kensico Cemetery in Valhalla. The headstone installed later inexplicably gives his birth year as 1905 when in fact it was 1903.

The public response to his death was phenomenal. Lou Gehrig's talent and especially his personal qualities were extolled in the editorial sections of many newspapers, a place where names of baseball players are seldom found. A bronze bust and memorial plaque were placed in center field at Yankee Stadium. An army air base in Texas named its athletic field after him and a World War II Liberty ship carried his name. Phi Delta Theta, Gehrig's fraternity, established the Lou Gehrig award in 1955, given annually since to the major league player judged to best exemplify Gehrig's personal character and playing ability. Thus, in death he received a kind of public adulation denied him during life when sportswriters, while acknowledging his athletic prowess, regarded him as colorless and uninteresting.

To capitalize on the Gehrig interest, someone suggested to movie mogul Samuel Goldwyn that a movie be made of his life. Goldwyn, who knew nothing about baseball, growled in response, "If people want to see baseball, they should go to a ballpark." But his associates insisted he view a newsreel of Gehrig's farewell speech, and Goldwyn emerged sobbing, needing no further urging. The resulting movie, *Pride of the Yankees,* starred Gary Cooper, an obvious choice by virtue of his image as a quiet and thoroughly decent man. However, Cooper lacked both knowledge and skills related to baseball, necessitating considerable cinematic sleight of hand for credible action scenes. The movie was an immediate box office smash and was nominated for Academy Awards in a number of categories in 1942. When Cooper entertained troops during World War II, he was most often asked to recite the Gehrig farewell speech. The movie remains a perennial favorite on late night TV channels and was recently voted number two on the all-time list of baseball movies.

Eleanor never remarried, continuing a relatively quiet and dignified life as guardian of the Gehrig legend. She appeared at Yankee old-timer games,

Hall of Fame inductions, and fundraisers for the disease that had killed her husband. In 1976, 35 years after Lou's death and eight years before her own, she co-authored a touching remembrance, *My Luke and I*, which later formed the basis of a made-for-TV movie, *A Love Story: Lou and Eleanor Gehrig*. In her book, she answered a frequent question about her six years of wedded bliss followed by two years of pain, and then loneliness:

> *I would not have traded two minutes of the joy and the grief with that man for two decades of anything with another. Happy or sad, filled with great expectations or great frustrations, we had attained it for whatever brief instant that fate had decided. The most in life, the unattainable, and we were not star-crossed by it. We were blessed with it, my Luke and I.*

To the public, Lou Gehrig passed quickly into legendary status. This was partly because of his outstanding athletic abilities and records, of course, but some others could match these. It was also in part a reflection of his personal qualities—modesty, diligence, and commitment—that every parent wishes in a son and what people like to think as the best America can offer. But it was mainly his tragically premature death of a horrible disease that enshrined him among America's heroes. He personified A. E. Houseman's well-known poem, To an Athlete Dying Young, especially its fourth verse:

> *Eyes the shady night has shut*
> *Cannot see the record cut,*
> *And silence sounds no worse than cheers*
> *After earth has stopped the ears:*

Medical Perspectives

The basic defect in ALS is degeneration and ultimate death of certain nerve cells in the brain and spinal cord. These cells, called motor neurons, represent the essential lines of communication between the central nervous system and muscles, functioning specifically by carrying impulses or messages from the brain to the spinal cord and from the spinal cord to voluntary muscles (i.e., those under voluntary control) throughout the body. When motor neurons die, they cannot be replaced and the brain loses the ability to initiate and control muscular activity. ALS does not affect nerve cells involved in sensation, so touch, sight, sound, smell and other sensations are intact. Memory and intellectual ability are also unaffected by the disease, as are cardiac, gastrointestinal, and urinary functions (while these entail muscular activity, the muscles involved are a different type and not under voluntary control). Thus, the person afflicted with ALS has difficulty with any voluntary movement, including breathing, swallowing, and talking, but can perceive, understand, and think normally.

The early symptoms experienced by people ultimately diagnosed with ALS are nearly always subtle and usually dismissed as inconsequential. There may be occasional muscle stiffness or twitching, slight weakness in an arm or a leg, difficulty swallowing, or slurred speech. A fairly common initial complaint among men is difficulty buttoning the shirt or tying the necktie. As the disease progresses, muscle weakness spreads to other areas of the body and then, when the deterioration of motor neurons is complete, there is total paralysis of the involved muscles. When muscles become nonfunctional, they undergo atrophy or wasting. In late stages of the disease, the major problems are nutritional (because of the inability to swallow) and respiratory (because of involvement of chest muscles and diaphragm, limiting breathing).

There are no specific diagnostic tests for ALS. The diagnosis can only be made by physical examination by a skilled and experienced examiner and by excluding other possible causes of muscle weakness. The course is downhill, usually at a fairly rapidly progressive rate, with death typically three to five years after diagnosis. In very rare cases, there may be a spontaneous arrest of the disease that can last five or ten years or even longer. When death comes, the usual cause is respiratory failure.

When Lou Gehrig was diagnosed with ALS in 1939, very few had ever heard of the disease; hence, its common designation as "Lou Gehrig's disease," a name that persists to this day. However, more recently nearly everyone knows of someone with ALS and many prominent people have been victims, including among others Senator Jacob Javits, actor David Niven, singer Dennis Day, and the subject of the long-running best seller *Tuesdays with Morrie*. These circumstances suggest that the disease may be increasing in frequency but most authorities agree that any apparent increase is likely due to better diagnostic abilities and that the actual incidence is not changing. The population frequency in the United States has been estimated anywhere between two and eight cases per 100,000 population and about 5,000 new cases are diagnosed each year. Men are affected slightly more often than women.

A small fraction of ALS cases, no more than 5 or 10%, seem to have a familial relationship, suggesting that some sort of genetic abnormality is responsible. However, the vast majority of ALS victims have no family history of the disease. Though there has been much research over many years, the cause of the disease or even its predisposing factors remain unknown. When the cause of a disease is unknown, there are usually a number of theories, a situation certainly true in the case of ALS.

One attractive theory involves some sort of environmental factor, especially a toxin, as responsible. However, in spite of concerted searching, no such common factor has been identified. Further, except for an isolated Pacific island where ALS seems to be unusually common, the frequency is essentially the same in different populations and ethnic groups throughout the world, which argues against any environmental contaminant as the cause. Another factor theorized is some type of infection or an unusual reaction to infection. Again, however, the constant distribution makes an infectious cause unlikely and extensive testing has failed to identify any antibody or other blood constituent characteristic of ALS. Yet another cause suggested is some sort of nutritional deficiency, but no evidence supporting a dietary origin has been found.

Another possible cause under consideration is a condition known as autoimmunity, a state in which an individual produces antibodies or other immune substances against his or her own body constituents. Rheumatoid arthritis and systemic lupus erythematosus are examples of diseases known to have an autoimmune basis. However, no immune substance has been identified in cases of ALS and, moreover, extensive treatment trials with cortisone-like drugs (to which autoimmune diseases typically respond, at least to some extent) have proven universally unsuccessful.

One of the more promising lines of research currently focuses on glutamate, an amino acid that normally acts as a neurotransmitter or chemical messenger in the brain. Glutamate levels appear to be higher than normal in the cerebrospinal fluid of at least some ALS patients and, moreover, artificially raising brain and spinal cord glutamate levels in animals seems to lead to increased death of motor neurons, an effect reminiscent of what is seen with ALS. However, even if elevated glutamate proves to be some sort of common feature of the disease, the essential question of what causes glutamate levels to be elevated remains problematic.

Because the cause of ALS is unknown, the only treatments are those directed toward symptoms. Drugs can be given to ease muscle cramps, decrease saliva production, or aid in sleeplessness or depression. Braces can help a victim remain ambulatory when muscles used in walking lose their function. Vacuum aspiration instruments can aid in handling excessive oral secretions that cannot be swallowed. A feeding tube placed in the stomach can maintain nutritional status when swallowing is impossible. The most serious involvement usually is when the muscles of respiration are affected, and respiratory failure is the usual cause of death. Studies have found that artificial ventilation at night early in the course seems to improve quality of life and delay respiratory failure.

In the early 1990s, the Food and Drug Administration, the branch of the U. S. government concerned with drug evaluation, authorized release of riluzole (Rilutek™), the first drug intended specifically for treatment of ALS. Riluzole lowers glutamate levels, decreasing damage to neurons from glutamate toxicity, and clinical trials have shown it to be associated with prolongation of survival for several months in ALS victims.

In the 70 years since Lou Gehrig manifested the disease that caused his premature death, a disease with which his name is inextricably linked, there has been much research directed toward unraveling the mysteries of ALS and trying to find effective treatments. Unfortunately, however, the cause of the disease remains unknown and its course and outcome are not greatly different today than they have always been. Someone who contracts ALS today might live a few months longer than Gehrig did, because of better supportive care and perhaps because of the new drug, riluzole. However, he or she will still die of the disease, after a protracted and discouraging course.

SOURCES

Eig Jonathon. *Luckiest Man: The Life and Death of Lou Gehrig.* Simon and Schuster, New York, 2005.

Gehrig Eleanor, Durso Joseph. *My Luke and I.* Thomas Y. Cromwell Company, New York, 1976

Robinson Ray. *Iron Horse: Lou Gehrig in His Time.* W.W. Norton & Company, New York, 1990.

www.baseball-reference.com. Accessed Augugst 26, 2007

www.alsa.org. Accessed September 22, 2007

CHAPTER 9

JEAN HARLOW AND CHRONIC KIDNEY DISEASE

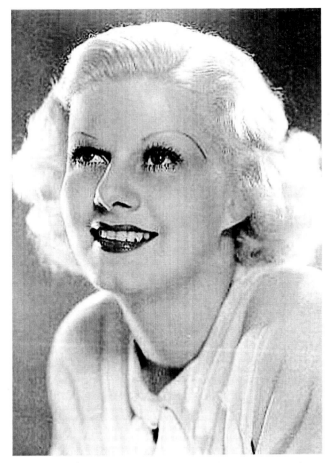

Figure 9.1 Jean Harlow (née Harlean Carpenter)

She was the original blonde bombshell, the first in a long line of flaxen-haired sex symbols that would eventually include Betty Grable, Jayne Mansfield, Madonna, and of course Marilyn Monroe. Her life was run—many would say ruined—by a domineering, overweening mother whose name she took as her own: Jean Harlow. She found her way into movies almost by accident and, lacking any experience or education in acting, her only credential was her incredible physical characteristics. In rather short order, she became a superstar and over time she developed a flair for comedy roles. She played roles opposite virile and dashing men like Clark Gable, Spencer Tracy, and Cary Grant, but her three marriages each involved weak and passive individuals, and had predictably sad outcomes. In fact, her relations with men generally, not only husbands but also lovers, agents, and managers, reflected her rather poor ability to judge character. At the height of her fame, when she was only 26, she became ill with the end-stage of chronic kidney disease and died within a few days. Nowadays kidney failure is amenable to treatment by dialysis or kidney transplant, but in those days its outcome was universally fatal.

Biography

S. D. (Skip) Harlow, a successful real estate broker in turn-of-the-century Kansas City, both indulged and dominated his wife and their only child, a daughter named Jean, just as Jean would later control her daughter. Harlow wanted grandchildren and he typically got what he wanted, so he pushed his daughter into marrying a young dentist, Mont Clair Carpenter. The couple moved into one of grandfather's houses and within a year or two Jean obligingly became pregnant. When she delivered, on March 3, 1911, the new grandfather was initially disappointed that it was a girl, but his feeling soon faded and he became even more indulgent than he had been with his daughter. The new baby was given the name Harlean Harlow Carpenter but her mother ever after referred to Harlean as "the Baby" or "Baby," names that friends adopted as well.

For Mother Jean, as she now styled herself, giving birth became the central feature of her existence: "There is nothing else in my life worth talking about because there is nothing else in my life." Moreover, in a stinging denial of basic biology, she asserted, "She was always all mine." Dr. Carpenter, having served his purpose, was quietly pushed into the background. His wife viewed him as dull and stodgy and had never cared much for him anyway. In 1922, she was granted a divorce and the following year she and the Baby (now 11 years old) moved to Hollywood where Mother Jean hoped to find a movie career. She was pretty enough but, at age 34, her prospects of breaking into movies were anything but favorable.

Nevertheless, she continued to seek her fortune in films, while enrolling her daughter in the Hollywood School for Girls where she came in contact with daughters of the great and near-great of the movie industry. Classmates recalled the 12-year-old Harlean as advanced well beyond her years, in both appearance and outlook. Her figure was stunning, her skin a perfect pink marble, her eyes a gorgeous green, and topping it all was a mop of real tow hair.

After two years of being supported by alimony and a subsidy from Grandfather Skip, Mother Jean faced a dilemma. Grandfather's generosity had run out and he ordered his daughter to bring Harlean home or be disinherited. Reluctantly, Mother Jean chose the former and she and Baby returned to dull and stifling Kansas City. Harlean was enrolled in one and then another private school and the next summer went to a camp in Michigan. It was here that she came down with scarlet fever and her mother rushed to her side, spending several weeks caring for her and, in a typical melodramatic description, saving Baby's life when all others had given up. On a stopover in Chicago on the way home, Mother Jean met Marino Bello, an Italian immigrant who charmed women with his dyed hair, waxed moustache, and hand kissing. It was a relationship that would exert lasting influences, none of them good, on mother and daughter.

The relationship between mother and daughter was by now well set and would continue unchanged for the rest of their lives. Mother Jean, while professing love and self-sacrifice, really was motivated by an overarching need to control. The daughter seems to have regarded her mother as an idol, something to be worshipped, and bent herself to her mother's every wish. Two notes written by Harlean, the first on her eighth birthday and the second 16 years later on the last Mother's Day of her life, were remarkably similar:

> *Dearest dearest Mother,*
> *Your gift was the sweetest of all. The little bracelet you gave*
> *me is to bind our love still tighter than it is, if that is possible.*
> *For I love you better than anything that ever its name was*
> *heard of.*
> *Please know that I love you better than ten lives.*
> *Yours forever into eternalty (sic).*
>
> *Your Baby*

> *Dearest of all mothers,*
> *This is Mother's Day to lots of People, but to me it's God's*
> *loveliest gift to humanity. You are God's finest conception of*

motherhood and I will always be eternally grateful He
allowed me the privilege of belonging to you.
I love you for now and forever.

Me

In 1926, Mother Jean convinced her father to let her enroll Harlean in Ferry Hall, an all-girl academy in Lake Forest, Illinois. Ferry Hall had a good reputation, but Jean's real motive was that her newfound Italian gigolo, Marino Bello, lived and worked in the vicinity. Harlean made quite an impression at the school. A classmate many years later had vivid recollections of her: "Flawless skin; the blondest hair, and it wasn't dyed; figure beautifully balanced, a great pair of legs, and a wonderful smile." She went on a blind date with Charles McGrew II from Lake Forest Academy, the male equivalent of Ferry Hall, and it was love at first sight. Their relationship blossomed and on September 21, 1927, they drove to Waukegan and were married by a justice of the peace. Harlean was 16 and Chuck was 20; when he turned 21 two months later he received $200,000, the first installment on a substantial inheritance.

The newlyweds quickly settled into a life that resembled something F. Scott Fitzgerald might write: riotous living, one party after another, and nonstop drinking. Chuck clearly was in the early stages of alcoholism. Harlean, ever the dutiful wife wanting to please, joined him in heavy drinking bouts and tried, not always successfully to keep up with him. In January 1928 they traveled by ship from New York to Los Angeles via the Panama Canal and took up residence in Beverly Hills. The couple fit in well in California and their life seemed happy, except for the drinking binges. Chuck regarded his wife as sensitive and intelligent and he treated her well. He made some attempts at finding a job, but they were not very serious ones for, after all, his inheritance relieved him of any real need to work.

It was at this time that something happened quite by chance, but it represented a certain historical significance. Harlean gave a friend a ride to Fox Studios for an appointment and, while waiting for the friend, she was seen by three Fox executives. They were taken with her and asked if she had any interest in trying to get into movies. She replied negatively, which was truthful for, in contrast to her mother, she had not been bitten with the movie bug. The executives regarded the response as a cute ploy, and they summoned a secretary to type a letter of introduction to Fox and the Central Casting Bureau. Harlean thanked them, put the letter in her purse, and forgot about it. However, a few weeks later, her friend who had witnessed the affair bet she wouldn't have the nerve to follow through, and Harlean did just that, for the sole purpose of winning the wager. Her visit to Central

Casting was brief and perfunctory, and all she really did was to leave her name. The name she decided to leave, on an impulse, was her mother's: Jean Harlow. Subsequently, she received several telephone invitations, all of which she declined, for she really had little interest in a movie career. However, her mother, who by now had married the Italian stallion and moved to Los Angeles, literally ordered her to accept the next offer. Ever the obedient daughter, Baby took work as an extra in a silent film about prison life, *Honor Bound,* released in 1928. There were more extra jobs, usually paying five or ten dollars a day, and by year-end she had progressed to bit parts, sometimes as "Harlean Carpenter" but increasingly as "Jean Harlow." She was recognized by many as possessing something special, with her striking appearance, a sweet kind of shyness, and an underlying sensuality.

While Jean's movie career was taking off, her marriage began to show signs of strain. Chuck McGrew was not particularly happy with a wife who spent most of her time on movie sets. He believed, undoubtedly correctly, that it was Mother Jean who was responsible for the rift between him and Harlean (as he still called her) by pressuring her daughter relentlessly, with the advice and encouragement of her charlatan-husband. Then a small glitch in Mother Jean's plans arose: Harlean discovered she was pregnant. The budding actress was overjoyed, believing that a child would save her marriage and allow her to cut back on her movie work. However, her mother told her a family could wait but her career could not, and the ever-dutiful daughter complied by undergoing an abortion. On June 11, 1929, Harlean and Chuck separated, and Mother Jean and Bello moved in with her. Later, the McGrews divorced.

Hollywood was in chaos in early 1929. Talking pictures had changed all the rules for actors, directors, and producers. Many who had experienced great success in silent films found they had little or no place in talkies. For Jean Harlow, who had been a bit player in a number of silent films, usually two-reelers, the turmoil presented an opportunity. Howard Hughes, a lanky, 23-year-old Texan was spending his father's fortune making *Hell's Angels,* a World War I aerial saga. It had started in 1927 as a silent film, but now Hughes decided to turn it into a sound movie. In reshooting the dramatic scenes, a problem quickly became apparent: the Norwegian actress who played the female lead had a heavy accent that was clearly unsuitable for the role of a sultry British woman. A replacement was needed, but Hughes was unable to recruit an established star, so he started searching for an unknown. Eventually, Jean Harlow's name came up. She took a quick screen test, for which she wore a tightly fitted evening gown, and the next morning, Hughes interviewed her for only a few minutes and hired her on the spot. And so a star was born.

But the road was hardly smooth. In the first place, Jean had had no formal acting education and her only experience was as a bit player. Moreover, her character in *Hell's Angels* was a sultry seductress, a role the simple and sweet actress had trouble playing in any sort of convincing way. Eventually, the filming was completed and the movie's premier on May 27, 1930 was extravagant even by Hollywood standards. Overall, the new star was reasonably well accepted by the public but the critics were merciless, *The New Yorker* reporting "Jean Harlow is plain awful." The actress went on a nationwide personal appearance tour that solidified her star status. She made a succession of movies over the next several months, working on loan from Hughes to M-G-M and Universal studios: *The Secret Six* (with Wallace Beery and Clark Gable), *The Iron Man* (with Lew Ayres), and *Public Enemy* (with James Cagney). She became type-cast as a sexy but unloving vamp who jumped from bed to bed—in one of her films the word "tramp" was first used to describe a woman—but these characteristics not really consistent with her actual personality. She was certainly not inhibited as far as sex was concerned and she had no reluctance in showing off her attention-getting physical characteristics. But at heart she was sweet and almost childlike, with an air of naiveté, and she had an even disposition of a type seldom seen in Hollywood stars. A writer once characterized her as "a regular girl with no vanity whatsoever—and no feeling about the sensation she created wherever she went."

Although her acting abilities remained problematic, Jean Harlow quickly replaced Clara Bow ("the It girl"), joining Greta Garbo, Rosalind Russell, and Myrna Loy as superstar actresses of the 1930s. The factor mainly responsible for Jean's rapid rise to stardom was, of course, her physical features. She was not very tall—only 5 feet 2 or 3 inches—but her figure was perfect, her legs shapely, and her skin flawless. However, it was her hair that made the greatest impression. She and Mother Jean would claim occasionally that it was natural, but no one believed them. In fact, to be a platinum blonde required hours each week with washes consisting of peroxide, ammonia, chlorine bleach, and commercial laundry soaps. This regimen left her hair brittle and difficult to shape, so it was necessary to apply oils and moisturizers and pin-curl or finger-wave it nearly every night. She also had to take precautions to avoid sun exposure. She did at least one film as a redhead and a couple as a brunette but it was a platinum blonde—a term first used in connection with her—that she would always be remembered.

Reviews of her acting, at least in the first several years, were pretty much uniformly negative. However, gradually the critics began to warm to her, finding that she did have some positive attributes. Beginning with no instruction or experience, she worked hard at improving and she was not devoid of talent. One of her strong points was an almost-photographic memory, giving her an ability to learn lines quickly. The most important step in her becoming a respected actress came when she was finally able to move away from the shameless hussy roles she had been cast in—and which she resented—and get parts she thought were more like her true self. In 1933 she was cast in *Dinner at Eight,* based on a long-running Broadway play and, in working with the well known comedienne Marie Dressler, Jean found her own natural abilities in comedy. The director, George Cukor, said, "I don't think you can teach people how to be funny. You can make suggestions about how to speak a line or get a laugh, but it has to be in them. Harlow played comedy as naturally as a hen lays an egg."

As her career moved to the stratosphere of superstardom, Baby's personal life continued its rocky road, with most of the bumps reflecting Mother Jean's incessant meddling. After separating from Chuck McGrew, the actress had several short-term affairs and then on June 21, 1932 she made the incredible announcement that she and Paul Bern would marry. Bern, an M-G-M studio executive, seemed the most unlikely candidate to wed his studio's hottest property. Twice her age, he was viewed as anything but romantic. To be sure, he had squired Harlow and other starlets around Hollywood, but his role seemed more that of a father figure. Some questioned his sexual orientation. The wedding took place on July 2 and almost immediately there were suggestions of problems. Nearly everyone involved would agree later that the marriage was never consummated. Nine weeks after the wedding, while Jean was staying overnight with friends, Bern would be found, naked and with a fatal gunshot wound to his head, in their home. The sad affair quickly morphed into a scandal that dwarfed even Hollywood's standards. There was a coroner's inquest that produced wild and lurid suggestions—that Bern was homosexual, that he was obsessed with obscure sexual practices, that he was impotent and/or had an underdeveloped sex organ, and even that Jean had killed him or arranged his murder. In spite of intensive study at the time and extensive speculation over the succeeding three-quarters of a century, there seem to be no reliable answers about Paul Bern's death.

Jean seemed prostrate with grief at Bern's funeral, but in only a few days she returned to work. She had several affairs, including an especially notable one with prizefighter Max Baer, and by a year after Bern's death the widow was actively looking for another mate. This one had to be ready, willing, and able—the last especially important in view of the unconsummated Bern marriage. Baby found her man in Hal Rosson, a cameraman who had filmed Jean in several pictures, and the two had always seemed to have a good rapport. In eerie similarities with Bern, Rosson was an old M-G-M hand and nearly twice the age of his bride. Friends had no questions, however, about his sexual orientation or performance. Many believed the marriage was promoted, perhaps even ordered, by the studio to offset any pending scandal arising from Jean's dalliance with Max Baer. The actress told reporters, "I know it's trite but I want to go on record that ours is one Hollywood marriage that will last." Last it did—for a total of 7 months and 17 days, until they formally separated. Shortly afterwards, they were divorced. Jean said, "We simply were not meant for each other." Hal refused to say anything, except to blame the "greedy, voracious prison keepers," Mother Jean and Bello. It was the Baby's third and final marriage.

Baby's last major relationship was with William Powell, an established Hollywood star who had been married twice, most recently to actress Carole Lombard. Powell, 18 years Jean's senior, was tall and handsome, in contrast to her last two husbands, and some thought he resembled the father from whom Baby had been separated at an early age. The couple worked together in *Reckless* and they were seen frequently in each other's company. The relationship was probably the most normal of Jean's several amorous affairs and the pair undoubtedly loved each other. Jean gushed ecstatically, "I never thought this would happen to me." But there was a hitch. She wanted desperately to marry and have children, but Powell was reluctant, saying they had both had unpleasant experiences with marriage. Jean hung on to the relationship, apparently hoping something would change. She began drinking excessively and on one occasion, bolstered by liquor, she confronted the person she and everyone else knew was really the cause of all her problems, past and present: her mother who had driven her to stardom against her wishes, wrecked her marriages, and squandered her money. But when she sobered up, she reverted to type as a docile, submissive daughter. She took up with a publisher who had come to Hollywood to sell film rights, while continuing the relationship with Powell.

In March 1937, M-G-M scheduled Harlow and Powell to make *The World's Our Oyster*, but a few weeks later the project was shelved and Jean switched to *Saratoga*, a racetrack romance, as a substitute for Joan Crawford. Filming began in March. It was the 22nd film in which Jean Harlow had star billing. It would be the last, though of course no one knew it at the time.

Illness and Death

The Baby had had several medical encounters during her 26 years but not very much is known about them, probably because of Mother Jean's tendency to use different doctors and thereby prevent anything resembling complete records. She had entered Good Samaritan Hospital on several occasions, twice for abortions (in 1932 and 1936 to interrupt pregnancies fathered by Charles McGrew and probably William Powell, respectively) and once in 1933 for an appendectomy.

Most biographers date the clear onset of Jean's deteriorating health to dental problems in early 1937. She complained of severe toothache and her dentist recommended removing her impacted wisdom teeth. He advised the extractions be done one at a time, but Mother Jean was adamant in insisting all be pulled at the same sitting and that the procedure be done under general anesthesia. She arranged for a plastic surgeon, an ophthalmologist, and an anesthesiologist—but no dentist—to perform the extractions on March 23 in Good Samaritan Hospital. It's not clear what happened during the procedure but there were complications, perhaps even cardiac arrest. However, the Baby eventually recovered and was discharged 18 days later. Shooting for *Saratoga* had already begun when Jean got to the set a few days later. Several of the crew thought she looked ill and she admitted she didn't feel well, the first time anyone could recall her voicing physical complaints. On Saturday, May 29, a friend thought she looked "pale and fragile" and the assistant director found her bloated enough to require a wardrobe re-fitting. In a scene with Walter Pidgeon that day, she doubled over with abdominal pain and he called to the director, "Baby's got a pain." She was sent to her dressing room to rest, but instead she changed her clothes and went to the set of *Double Wedding* to tell William Powell she was going to his mansion.

During that day and the next, the actress's condition seemed to worsen. She alternated between fever and chills and she took little or nothing by mouth. By Sunday evening, Powell was alarmed enough to call Mother Jean, who had taken a brief trip to Catalina Island. She hurried back the next morning and immediately assumed her usual role as commanding officer, ordering her daughter taken to their home and sending for Dr. Ernest Fishbaugh. Dr. Fishbaugh, an internist who had some previous dealings with the family, examined his patient on Monday evening the 31st, Memorial Day. He diagnosed a "severe cold" and a "stomach ailment," took some blood and urine samples, and assigned nurses from Good Samaritan Hospital to provide around-the-clock care. The next morning, Jean called the director to report. "I'm so sick I can't come to work." He assured her they would shoot around her until she felt better. No one on the crew was particularly alarmed, for Jean had occasionally caused delays in other filmings. Someone even suggested she might be on a drinking binge. But she was critically ill.

On Wednesday, Harlow complained of abdominal pain, vomited, and seemed to become delirious, at least intermittently. Dr. Fishbaugh, whose diagnosis at this point became cholecystitis (i.e., inflammation of the gall bladder), judged her too ill to transfer and he ordered special medical equipment to be sent from Good Samaritan. The home was probably equipped and staffed as well as most hospitals of that time. Then the Baby seemed to rally. The next day she sat up in bed and ate a little and Mother Jean announced the doctor had determined she was "out of danger." Studio executives even reported they expected her return to the *Saratoga* set on Friday or Monday. Many friends wanted to visit, but Mother Jean was in control and she refused most requests. Clark Gable, her co-star on *Saratoga*, was one of the few visitors allowed and he said later she was bloated to twice her normal size and when he bent forward to kiss her he smelled urine on her breath.

Mother Jean brushed aside suggestions that Baby should be hospitalized, saying "We are Christian Scientists." This statement later gave rise to a persistent myth that she was responsible for her daughter's death by denying her needed medical care. In fact, Jean Harlow probably received as good a level of medical care as existed at the time: her room was well equipped and she had continuous nursing care and physician visits at least once each day. Moreover, neither mother nor daughter had any actual connection with the Church of Christ, Scientist. The whole thing was a ploy to keep Baby under her mother's control. Using it, Mother Jean was able to refuse advice and offers of assistance, including movie mogul Louis B. Mayer's offer of his personal physician.

Over the next several days, as it became clear that Jean was not improving, even Mother Jean concluded that a change in doctors was needed. She called Dr. Leland Chapman, a junior associate of Dr. Fishbaugh, and begged him to take over the case. Chapman was reluctant to intrude on another doctor's patient, particularly when the doctor was a senior colleague. However, when one of the nurses on duty called and told him he was needed, he relented. Reviewing the records, especially the blood chemistry tests, he realized Jean had, not gall bladder inflammation as Dr. Fishbaugh had diagnosed, but chronic progressive disease of the kidneys that had reached the point where her kidney function was insufficient to maintain life. He said later that Fishbaugh was a good doctor who had simply made a wrong diagnosis in this instance. So while Fishbaugh remained the physician of record, Chapman took over the care of the patient. He reduced the volumes of fluids being administered intravenously, for her failing kidneys could not excrete urine well and the resulting fluid accumulation was the reason for her swelling. He probably also gave a diuretic in an effort to stimulate kidney function, but this was not likely be very effective, for kidney function by this point was past the point where it could be goaded into action.

By this time, Jean's blood was loaded with accumulating waste products of protein metabolism, mainly urea, and she had a condition known as uremia or uremic poisoning. Individuals with this condition, since their kidneys cannot rid them of metabolic waste products, tend to excrete small amounts of urea in sweat and expired air, giving the distinctive uriniferous odor many recognized pervading Jean's sick room. Uremia also results in altered states of consciousness, so affected people tend to sleep a great deal. In advanced stages, vision can be impaired. Thus, when William Powell first visited Jean on Sunday, June 6, she had difficulty recognizing him and could not tell how many fingers he held up. That evening, it was clear she was dying, and an ambulance transferred her to Good Samaritan Hospital. She was placed in an oxygen tent and given blood transfusions, presumably because of anemia, a common complication of chronic kidney disease. The following morning, following unsuccessful attempts to ventilate her artificially and surrounded by her doctors, nurses, and the ever-present Mother Jean, a bloated and semi-conscious Jean Harlow breathed her last. Virtually every newspaper reported her death in a front-page article, either that afternoon or the next morning.

Death was attributed to "acute nephritis" but based on the clinical picture, especially the probable presence of anemia, the cause was much more likely the chronic variety, specifically chronic glomerulonephritis. In this condition, the affected part of the kidney is primarily the glomeruli, the many small blood vessel structures involved in the first stage of filtering blood components to make urine. The disease likely had its origin in the episode of scarlet fever Harlean has experienced as a teenager at summer camp. Scarlet fever comes from streptococcal infections of the throat, and a few individuals experience a reaction to a "strep throat" that triggers the onset of glomerulonephritis. The condition smolders for many years, basically symptomless, while kidney function deteriorates progressively. Eventually, a critical point is reached when function is no longer adequate to the body's needs. Glomerulonephritis is usually accompanied by high blood pressure and it is somewhat curious that nothing is mentioned about her blood pressure in any of the medical records available.

The funeral, held on June 9 at Wee Kirk o' the Heather in Forest Lawn Memorial Park Glendale, was vintage Hollywood. All the celebrities were there: Clark Gable, Carole Lombard, Spencer Tracy, Myrna Loy, Norma Shearer, Wallace Beery, Lionel Barrymore, Robert Montgomery, Ronald Coleman, and the Marx Brothers, along with executives of all the major studios. William Powell was so grief-stricken he needed assistance to walk to the chapel. The corpse was dressed in a pink silk negligee she had worn in *Saratoga* and a platinum blonde wig (because her head had been shaved shortly before her death in preparation for drilling holes in the skull to relieve brain swelling, which was never done). There were more elaborate floral displays than anyone could remember in any previous Hollywood funeral. Scattered among the opulent flower arrangements were more modest bouquets from gaffers, grips, and other crewmembers, for the "ordinary people" with whom Jean Harlow worked had adored her. The service itself was brief: Jeanette MacDonald sang *Indian Love Call;* a Christian Scientist practitioner read from the 29th Psalm, recited the Lord's Prayer, and gave a eulogy lasting less than a minute; and Nelson Eddy sang *Ah, Sweet Mystery of Life.* It was all over in 38 minutes.

Mother Jean had one final ploy to spring. She issued a press statement, "As a shrine for the Baby, Bill Powell bought the room where she will lie forever." It was a lavish, marble-lined room in the Sanctuary of Benediction in Forest Lawn's Great Mausoleum and it contained two additional places, one for Mother Jean and the other presumably for Powell himself. Powell, of course, knew nothing about all this, but there was little he could do about it after the public announcement. When the bill for $30,000 (equivalent to about a half-million today) arrived later, he realized just how much he had been rooked.

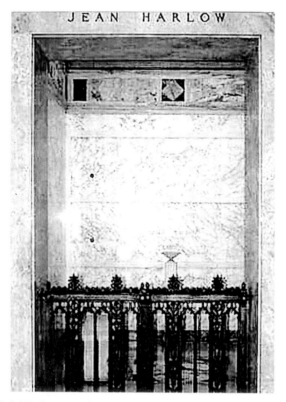

Figure 9.2 Harlow tomb, Great Mausoleum, Forest Park Glendale

Scarcely was the Baby in her place of final repose before all sorts of theories about her death sprang up. In addition to the argument mentioned previously that her mother in essence killed her by denying medical care, there were proposals that she had cancer, heart disease, and polio; was poisoned; and died of a botched abortion. One especially fanciful suggestion that is still widely held is that agents used to bleach her hair destroyed her kidneys. An especially scurrilous and wildly inaccurate book appeared in the 1960s and was to form the basis for a movie. Marilyn Monroe, in many ways Jean Harlow's legatee, was recruited for the part but after reading the script she turned it down flat.

The movie industry is notorious for not tarrying long with unpleasant situations. *Saratoga,* the movie Jean Harlow was doing at the time of her death, resumed after a short interval and, using creative editing and doubles for the deceased star's body and voice, it was released in late July. The critics gave it a mixed judgment but people flocked to see it and its gross income was the highest of any film that year.

The main characters in Jean Harlow's life also moved on, albeit in different ways and at different paces. Mother Jean, having ridded herself of the philandering and plundering Marino Bello two years earlier, found no role in the movie industry, so she moved to a home in the San Fernando Valley that she decorated as a shrine to her daughter. She also consulted psychics in efforts to contact Baby. In 1944 she married but two years later she divorced. For a time she ran an antiques shop in Palm Desert. Eventually, she settled in a small home on Beverly Glen Boulevard, the same street of the mansion that was her home during the glory days. In 1958, at the age of 69, she died of a heart attack, and so at last she took her place next to her beloved Baby in the Forest Lawn mausoleum.

William Powell, the last and probably truest love of Jean Harlow, was devastated with guilt and had difficulty getting over her death. He could not continue in movies and then he was diagnosed with rectal cancer. Following a two-year period of treatment and rehabilitation, both physical and mental, he returned to a very successful film career. Finally ready for a commitment, he married and had a long, happy, and productive life. At his death in 1984 at age 91, the spot reserved for him for eternity in the Forest Lawn mausoleum was totally ignored. It remains empty.

Medical Perspectives

The kidney, of which each person normally has two, is essential in maintaining health. Its principal function is that of excretion, the removal from the blood of waste products of metabolism, other unwanted materials, and excess water. Blood flow to the kidneys is enormous, amounting to about 200 liters each day, from which the kidney produces about 2 liters of urine. There are two main steps in this excretory function. Blood passes first through minute vascular structures called glomeruli (of which there are normally about a million) where water and waste products, but not solid materials like cells, diffuse from the blood. Then what has been filtered from the blood goes to the tubules where most of the water and electrolytes are reabsorbed back into the circulation and a few more substances are excreted, forming what we recognize as urine, which then passes into the bladder and ultimately outside the body. The process is complex and intricate, but absolutely essential in maintaining health. In addition to its excretory function, the kidney has several other important roles. It produces hormones that regulate three essential functions: blood pressure and volume, red blood cell production, and bone calcification.

The kidney possesses a phenomenal degree of reserve. A healthy person can remain healthy after losing one of his or her kidneys; as is well known, kidney donors do exactly this. In fact, people with kidney disease generally have little in the way of symptoms or signs until 85-90% of function is lost. Only when this critical level is reached will there be clinical evidence of impaired function.

Many different diseases can affect the kidney. Some are acute, with sudden onset and usually rapid course, such as most kidney infections. Acute kidney problems can occasionally be severe but they usually respond to appropriate therapy and leave little residual damage. Chronic diseases are more insidious in their onset and gradual in their course, but over time they can destroy or damage enough kidney tissue to lead to organ failure. Chronic kidney disease will be the focus of this discussion.

Historically, the name most connected with chronic kidney (or renal) disease is that of Richard Bright, an English physician of the early 19th century who gave the first clinical description and noted the association with protein in the urine. What came to be known as Bright's disease was originally assumed to be a single condition. However, it is now recognized that many different diseases affecting the kidney, both inherited and acquired, can be manifest in much the same way, and so the eponym has lost its original meaning. It is still used occasionally, more to honor Bright's contributions than for any specific diagnostic meaning.

The National Kidney Foundation estimates that 26 million Americans are presently living with some degree of chronic kidney disease. The vast majority lack symptoms and most are unaware of their condition. The three most common causes of chronic kidney disease, together accounting for 75% of cases, are diabetes (37%), hypertension (24%), and glomerulonephritis (16%). Considering only the most severe stage, 45-50% are due to diabetes and 25-30% to hypertension. Diabetes, a disease of carbohydrate (sugar) metabolism predisposes to arterial disease and the extensive blood vessel network of the kidney is frequently affected. The relation between hypertension (high blood pressure) and kidney disease is bi-directional in that hypertension can cause chronic kidney disease and chronic kidney disease can cause hypertension. Glomerulonephritis refers to a group of diseases causing damage to the glomerulus, the structure mainly responsible for initial filtering of blood; one such condition occurs as a reaction to infection with the streptococcus.

Five stages of chronic kidney disease, based chemical tests of kidney function, are recognized. The fifth and most advanced stage, called chronic kidney (or renal) failure or end-stage renal disease, affects an estimated half-million Americans presently. It is characterized by decreasing urine volume and progressively elevated blood levels of waste products of protein metabolism, especially urea (often called BUN for blood urea nitrogen) and creatinine. The state of high blood urea levels is called azotemia and when accompanied by lethargy and altered consciousness, the condition is known as uremia. There is usually high blood pressure, which (as noted previously) may be either primary or secondary. Body fluids increase, leading to a bloated and swollen appearance and perhaps difficulty breathing because of lung fluid accumulation. Along with urea and creatinine, potassium levels rise in the blood and may cause heart arrythmias. Blood calcium falls and calcium is leached from bone. A terminal event is often an acidic state in the blood because the failed kidney cannot rid the body of excessive acid.

Chronic kidney disease, unique in being the only disease covered by the federal Medicare program without regard to age, is increasing in frequency. The overall prevalence of stages 1-4 increased from 10% in 1988-1994 to 13.1% in 1999-2004. At least part of the increase reflects aging of the population and increased frequency of diabetes, hypertension, and obesity. There may also be some apparent increase related to better diagnosis. Until relatively recently, the most severe stage of chronic kidney disease (i.e., kidney failure or end-stage renal disease) was universally fatal, but advances over the last half-century or so have markedly improved this previously abysmal prognosis. These therapeutic advances, known collectively as renal replacement therapy, consist of two main treatments: dialysis and kidney transplantation.

Dialysis uses the principle of diffusion across a membrane to rid the body of undesired substances and excess water, diffusion occurring from the side of high concentration to that of lower amounts. In the case of kidney failure, metabolic waste products (e.g., urea) and other toxic substances (e.g., potassium) build up, but their blood levels fall as they diffuse from blood through the membrane to a fluid on the other side, in essence cleansing the blood of undesired and toxic materials which are then discarded with the dialyzing fluid. Blood volume can be regulated by this technique as well. Two different types of dialysis exist, hemodialysis and peritoneal dialysis.

Hemodialysis has a history going back to 19th century efforts to use the principle of dialysis to replace the kidney's excretory function. However, it was not until the 1940s that a clinically useful "artificial kidney" was developed. Many technical problems needed to be solved to enable blood to be pumped into the apparatus where it could be exposed to a membrane separating it from a fluid lacking the undesirable compounds, and then to pump the cleansed blood back into the person. Not least of these problems was that of vascular access, since the process must be repeated frequently. Initially, hemodialysis use was limited to acute, short-term conditions of kidney failure where the goal was to take care of the problem temporarily until the patient's kidneys recovered. For example, with significant and prolonged fall in blood pressure (such as shock from massive hemorrhage), the kidneys are not perfused with blood and they can shut down; similarly, acute kidney failure can result from any of several toxic drugs or other substances. In either instance, the damage is often temporary and, if the patient can be "tided over" for a few weeks, the kidney will eventually recover and resume normal function. Hemodialysis worked well for this purpose. However, acute kidney failure of this type is unusual, and most of the time kidney failure is chronic, meaning it follows a prolonged course and, more importantly, will never recover on its own.

In about 1960 a major technical advance made long term hemodialysis feasible: a permanent plastic shunt implanted by minor surgery between an artery and a vein, usually in the arm, permitting repeated vascular access. As a result of this technique and progressive advances in dialysis technology over the past 40 years, many people with chronic kidney failure have avoided inevitable death, at least in the near term (e.g., only half of patients starting dialysis survive for 3 years). Overall, however, the health and quality of life with dialysis, while far from perfect, has become reasonable. Dialysis centers, developed originally in hospitals, are now largely free-standing units; of an estimated 3600 facilities scattered throughout the United States today, only 260 are hospital-based. They are located throughout the country and the developed world, so that kidney failure patients are potentially able to travel quite freely. The National Kidney Foundation estimates that 341,000 Americans, about 70% of those with end-stage renal disease, are currently receiving regular dialysis (the rest have undergone kidney transplants).

The procedure of hemodialysis involves opening the vascular access and connecting it to the dialysis machine or artificial kidney. Each treatment requires about 4 hours, during which the subject reclines and reads, sleeps, or watches television. It is usually done three times per week Evidence exists that longer and/or more frequent treatments improve results, but the present program of thrice weekly for 4 hours each is a compromise with issues of cost and patient inconvenience. A relatively recent development, hemodialysis at home, offers potential for improved outcome, but it requires substantial motivation and assistance from knowledgeable caregivers, and cost remains a major problem.

Peritoneal dialysis uses the peritoneum, a membrane lining the abdominal cavity, to accomplish the same goal of cleansing the blood. A sterile solution containing important minerals and sugar (but no metabolic waste products) is run through a tube into the abdominal cavity, left for several hours, and then removed through the same tube and discarded. The process usually needs to be done about four times a day, but a continuous technique also exists. Peritoneal dialysis requires considerable patient motivation and even more time than hemodialysis, although being done at home makes it less expensive. It is also less efficient than hemodialysis in removing waste products. For these reasons peritoneal dialysis is being used less and less, although some kidney specialists regard it as a useful adjunct in treating early cases in which some kidney function remains.

The second major form of renal replacement therapy is kidney transplantation. Joseph E. Murray performed the first successful transplant in 1954 but it involved identical twins, finessing the problem of rejection of foreign tissue. The recipient was still alive in 2005. Murray continued working on transplantation between unrelated donors, and he was recognized by award of the Nobel Prize in Physiology or Medicine in 1990. The kidney is relatively easy to transplant technically and the major obstacle that needed to be overcome was rejection by the recipient's immune system. This became feasible in the 1960s with the development of increasingly effective immunosuppressive drug regimens. The mainstay of therapy involves cortisone-like drugs, typically prednisone, combined with (usually two) other agents that suppress the immune reaction by different means. Immunosuppressive drugs must be taken for the recipient's life and require fairly careful monitoring to maintain the relatively narrow balance between over- and underdosage. Long-term immunosuppressive drug treatment carries some risk of complications and a range of side effects, including increased risk of infections and even certain cancers, so careful follow-up care is essential.

Kidneys for transplantation may come from living donors (often a relative, which increases the likelihood of a close immunologic match) or from individuals who died very recently (called cadavers). The closer donor and recipient are matched on immunologic tests, including blood type and other immune characteristics, the better will the outcome be. Following transplantation, the donor must be monitored carefully because signs of rejection occur in 10-20% of cases during the first month or two postoperatively; this can sometimes be controlled with medical therapy, but occasionally the organ is non-functional and must be removed and replaced.

Statistics on kidney transplantation, because it is costly in both financial and human terms, are tabulated precisely and completely by an agency sponsored by the federal government, the Organ Procurement and Transplantation Network and the Scientific Registry of Transplant Recipients. In 2005, the most recent year for which figures are available, 16,072 patients underwent kidney transplantation, 60% from cadavers and 40% from living donors. The outcome varies somewhat with the source of the organ: overall patient survival at 1 and 5 years was 98% and 94%, respectively, with living donors and 95% and 81%, respectively, with cadaveric transplants. Of all the organs amenable to transplantation, the kidney is the one with which there is most experience and the best outcome. It is estimated that about 140,000 Americans are presently living with transplanted kidneys. Included in that number are several world-class professional athletes, some of whom returned to their sports after having undergone kidney transplants.

When chronic kidney disease reaches stage 5 (i.e., kidney failure or end-stage renal disease), something must be done for the individual to survive. Almost always, dialysis is the first step, and often it represents the preferred choice for continuing therapy. Patients who are older and/or have other significant medical problems are usually better served with long-term dialysis, avoiding the risks of major surgery and immunosuppression, whereas younger and healthier subjects represent better candidates for transplantation. In choosing between the two modes of renal replacement therapy, in addition to age and medical status, factors of convenience and efficacy are often influential. The situation represents a trade-off in that dialysis is less convenient, requiring at least 12 hours each week spent connected to a machine, whereas transplantation carries the risk and short-term disability of major surgery and some continuing potential problem with immunosuppression. However, when transplantation is feasible, it is generally less intrusive in the long run, allows better mobility and quality of life, and probably yields somewhat better results. Transplantation is limited by the fact that there are fewer kidneys available than needed, even by suitable candidates: according to the transplant network data, the waiting list for renal transplants numbered 62,294 at the end of 2005, nearly four times the number of transplants done per year.

As noted earlier, the kidney has several important functions in addition to excretion and these require attention in those undergoing renal replacement therapy, either dialysis or transplantation. Anemia often occurs because of a lack of the kidney hormone (erythropoietin) that stimulates red blood cell production; most kidney failure patients need to take a synthetic form of this hormone. Another kidney hormone, derived from vitamin D, also needs to be taken to stabilize calcium levels and maintain bone health. The kidney being a major site of excretion of drugs, medications indicated to treat conditions other than kidney disease must be monitored carefully. Additionally, careful attention to acid-base status is needed.

While modern treatments of chronic kidney disease, especially renal replacement therapy, have greatly improved outcomes, the condition remains an important health risk. In 2004, it was the ninth leading cause of death in the United States, with a mortality rate (unadjusted for age and other factors) of 14.5 deaths per 100,000 population. By comparison, in the year Jean Harlow died, 1936, the comparable figure was 83.2 deaths per 100,000 population.

What would have been Jean Harlow's fate had she been born 30 or 40 years later than was actually the case? In the first place, her streptococcal throat infection as a teenager would be treated with penicillin, which would have probably prevented development of glomerulonephritis. Even if it did not, or if the cause of her kidney failure were something else, when kidney failure became evident, she would have been started on dialysis and, in view of her age, probably would have undergone a transplant operation fairly promptly. Thus, there is a strong likelihood that her outcome, in terms of long-term and reasonably normal existence, would be good and her movie star career could have gone on much longer.

SOURCES

Stenn David. *Bombshell: The Life and Death of Jean Harlow.* Bantam Doubleday Dell. New York. 1993

Golden Eve. *Platinum Girl: The Life and Legends of Jean Harlow.* Abbeville Press. New York. 1991.

Coresh J, Selvin E, Stevens LA. Prevalence of chronic kidney disease in the United States. *JAMA* 2007;298:2038-47.

www.kidney.org. Accessed April 2, 2008.

www.ustransplant.org. Accessed April 5, 2008

CHAPTER 10

EVA PERON AND CANCER OF THE CERVIX

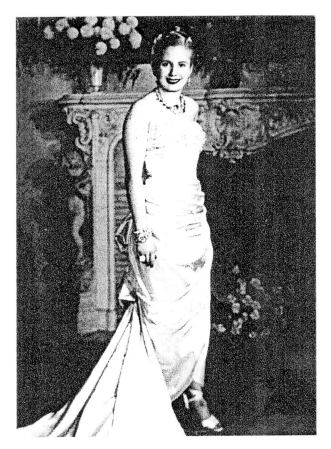

Figure 10.1 Eva Perón, in all her glory
(With permission from Pitkin RM *ACOG Clinical Review* 2004; 6: 11-6)

Eva Perón rose from the most humble of beginnings to become arguably the most powerful female political figure of the 20th century. Born to a single mother in rural Argentina, she became a star of radio and movies and then, through marriage to a man destined for the presidency of the country, she acquired vast political power. An ambitious program of social action earned her the veneration of the working classes and the underprivileged, but repressive ways of dealing with any kind of dissent brought controversy. In any case, during a meteoric career in the late 1940s, she was one of the world's best-known and most glamorous women. Early death conferred a kind of martyr status, at least as far as her adoring masses were concerned, and her legend was enhanced further during the 1980s by release of the immensely popular Andrew Lloyd Weber musical *Evita*. She died of cancer of the cervix, a disease that has come under control, at least in developed countries, by screening programs leading to early case finding. Now, a vaccine against a virus that causes the disease offers the possibility of eliminating it.

<u>Biography</u>

On May 7, 1919, in the dusty, squalid village of Los Toldos on the vast, treeless Argentine *pampa,* an unmarried woman named Juana Ibarguren gave birth to her fifth child, all fathered by Juan Duarte, a married man. The baby was given the name Maria Eva and, after the father died in 1926, both mother and children assumed his surname. Life was hard on the Argentine plain, especially for children born out of wedlock. It was certainly not unusual for a man to take a mistress, but the conservative, Catholic culture of Argentina viewed the offspring of such unions with special disdain. Much later, Eva would say that the hardships and cruelty she experienced as a child were what fired her commitment to social justice for the downtrodden masses.

Eva attended school through six primary grades, first in Los Toldos and then in Junín, a somewhat larger town where the family moved when she was 11. Her academic record was average. Teachers and students remembered her as a thin, pale brunette whose most memorable physical feature was her large, expressive, brown eyes. In manner, she was quiet, sensitive, and withdrawn. At age 14, she was given a small part in a school play, and suddenly her life had purpose. She announced she would be an actress, and a year later she went to Buenos Aires in pursuit of her dream. Buenos Aires was then one of the world's most cosmopolitan cities and it must have been daunting for a 15-year-old girl from the hinterlands and alone. She made the rounds of theaters, agents, and acting companies, but jobs were few and very far between. Probably—although her supporters would deny it vehemently—she became involved with a succession of lovers, generally of increasing social and economic status, who provided food and housing. Gradually persistence began to pay off for Eva, or Evita as she began to use as a stage name. Her big break came in 1939, just before her 20th birthday, when she landed a part in a radio drama. This led to a succession of acting jobs, mainly in radio but also in movies, culminating in January 1943 with a weekly radio series in which she played the roles of great women in history. It was wildly successful and it made Evita a national celebrity.

At a benefit for earthquake victims a year later, Evita arranged to meet Colonel Juan Domingo Perón, a handsome widower who was recognized as a rising star in the military government of Argentina. Her interest in him was no surprise, for he held two important posts simultaneously, Secretary of War and Secretary of Labor and Social Security. It was apparently love at first sight and before long Perón moved into an apartment next to hers. Their affair may have caused some discomfort among some of the conservative Army officers but it certainly enhanced Evita's celebrity status. Her radio salary increased and she won a part in a new movie, one that required her to bleach her hair. Ever after, she would remain a blonde.

Eva quickly became very influential in the politics of the movement becoming known as Perónism. She sensed the vast untapped source of political power latent in the hordes of poor people pouring into Buenos Aires and she knew of their frustrations with past electoral fraud that had deprived them of any say in the government. Undoubtedly at Eva's urging, Perón as Secretary of Labor and Social Security decreed a minimum wage, improved working condition, and, in the most popular move of all, established the *aguinaldo,* the wage for the 13th month given to every worker just before Christmas. Employers and other members of the landed aristocracy did not like these initiatives, but the actions made Perón extremely popular with the masses. Perón also extended his authority to the labor unions, rooting out Communist influences, and making them subservient to him. In recognition of his popular standing, he was appointed Vice-President, the second most powerful position in the country.

In the early months of 1945, Perón's rise to power hit a snag. Support of the Army, critical in Argentina, began to weaken because of feelings he was becoming too powerful. There was also lingering concern about his domestic situation and the power wielded by his mistress. Another factor was the persistent stain of fascism and even Nazism. Perón had served as military attaché to Italy and he made no secret of his admiration for Mussolini and perhaps for Hitler as well. Argentina remained neutral until the very end of World War II but, as the defeat of the Axis powers became inevitable, this admiration became a liability. In October, things came to a head and Perón

151

was forced to resign and incarcerated. Eva contacted many labor leaders friendly (and indebted) to Perón and they called a general strike and organized a massive march on Buenos Aires. On October 17—a day that would become the holiest day of Perónism—the government backed down, releasing Perón and restoring him to his offices.

Immediately after the triumph of October 17, Juan Domingo Perón and Maria Eva Duarte were married and they then plunged into a campaign for the office of President. The handsome and dashing colonel and his beautiful celebrity wife traveled the length and breadth of Argentina, always giving their message of welfare for the downtrodden masses and social justice for the working people, at the expense of the landowning aristocracy. It was a message that resonated well, for when the election results were announced in late March, Perón had won a smashing victory. At his side when he took the oath as 29th President of Argentina was Señora Eva Duarte de Perón and it soon became clear that she would be a full partner in the new venture. She immersed herself in the business of governing in a way never seen before or, for that matter, since. Although she had no official position, she could be found at her office in a government building from early morning to evening, receiving delegations of workers wanting salary increases, women wanting relief from the *machismo* culture, politicians wanting some kind of favor, and so on. Virtually everyone got what he or she came for. She could be generous in granting all these requests because the Argentine economy was booming. Argentina had meat and grain to supply a world devastated by war, a war in which Argentina lost nothing and gained much, and nationalization of transportation and utilities added to government coffers.

Late in her working day, she met with common, ordinary people who came requesting some urgent need like housing or food or treatment of a sick child. She would flit from one petitioner to another, scribbling a note or barking an order to an aide, touching and looking into the eyes of each supplicant, and then handing each a crisp new 50-peso banknote. An American reporter, on seeing her in one of these daily sessions, likened it to watching someone playing 50 chess games simultaneously.

Eva was the public face of Perónism and she seemed to be everywhere—opening factories, touring slums, comforting those who were ill or injured, and standing as godparent to a couple's seventh son. Moreover, she projected a very glamorous image, and this entailed clothes and jewelry on a staggeringly lavish scale. Such ostentatious displays might seem detrimental to the image of "The Lady of Hope," as she styled herself, to the millions mired in poverty, but Eva dismissed such concerns. Since she came from that class herself, she argued, seeing her dressed richly meant they could hope for something similar and this would actually hearten the poor. The reasoning might seem contrived, but it apparently worked. Her instincts rarely betrayed her in her dealings with the people.

Evita's glamorous image received worldwide exposure when the Spanish dictator, Franco, named her to receive the Grand Cross of Isabel the Catholic. She took advantage of the opportunity to make a grand tour of Europe, starting with a series of lavish receptions in Spain and then in Italy where she had a papal audience. She also toured France and Switzerland, where her reception was rather more mixed, before returning home two months later. Eva Perón had clearly arrived on the world stage, as evidenced by her image appearing twice on the cover of *Time* magazine, in 1947 by herself and in 1951 with Juan.

Evita—the familiar name she encouraged all to call her—was adored and worshipped as a saint by the Argentine working class. But the feeling was by no means unanimous. The upper classes, what she call the oligarchy, detested her and the social justice gospel she preached, a gospel which, to be sure, deprived them of their formerly-complete control of government and society. Others were concerned about Evita and Perónism, not so much because their wealth was threatened, but because of repressive measures in stifling anything that looked like dissent. Within a year of Perón's inauguration as President, he or his wife owned or controlled all four Buenos Aires radio stations, owned outright two newspapers in the capital city, and, through the Ministry of Information, exercised censorship over all radio stations in the country. Any media outlets that seemed in the least critical of the government were likely to find themselves harassed by government inspectors seeking the slightest infraction of labor laws or working condition regulations. Sometimes, opposition newspapers or radio stations might be attacked by street gangs, and the police response could be slow. However, if there was concern, both in Argentina and the rest of the world, about civil liberties, it was clearly a minority position.

Although there seemed to be controversy surrounding most of Evita's doings, in some things she seemed above reproach to any but the most critical eye. One of these was women's suffrage. Bills to give women the right to vote had been introduced in the Argentine legislature a number of times since the early part of the century, but none had ever been enacted. Eva persuaded her husband to make women's suffrage a priority on the Perónism agenda but, while other priorities became law, the all-male legislature let this matter languish. After a year or two of this, Evita took things into her own hands. She marched into the legislative chamber and, with the galleries by pre-arrangement packed with women, announced she would not leave until the bill was taken up. It passed quickly and became law with Perón's signature.

Another relatively non-controversial accomplishment was the Maria Eva Duarte de Perón Social Aid Foundation, established in July 1948 and changed two years later to the Eva Perón Foundation. Conceived as an instrument of social justice rather than of charity, it had a broad mandate to support all kinds of educational activities, provide housing and food to the needy, build hospitals and clinics, and do just about anything its founder wished. Its resources quickly grew to enormous proportions because businesses and citizens alike contributed, a portion of the government lottery was earmarked for it, and the legislature made direct appropriations. Labor union members who questioned the "voluntary" donation of two days' pay each year were reminded that it was the Foundation's director who would rule on their future requests for salary increases and improved working conditions. Business that hesitated to make their "voluntary" donation found themselves subjected to frequent inspections of their compliance with various ordinances covering cleanliness, sanitation, and working conditions. There was never any accounting of the Foundation's receipts or expenditures. Eva brushed aside any questions about such matters by saying she wanted to help the poor, not be an accountant. There was probably some graft involved and some of the money may well have gone to support the lavish lifestyle of Eva and her family, but undoubtedly much good was done. The number of hospitals in Argentina doubled between 1946 and 1949 (many of them, of course, bearing the Perón name), and hundreds of schools and homes for unwed mothers, orphans, and the aged were built.

Evita's high public profile might suggest that she was the real power and her husband merely a figurehead. She, however, was always deferential, almost obsequious, in her public pronouncements, seeming to minimize her own role and glorifying that of her husband. Asked once how she might be remembered, she replied "All I ask is that history note there was a woman alongside General Perón, who took to him the hopes and needs of the people, and her name was Evita." The truth undoubtedly lies between these two extremes. The relationship between the two Peróns, while complex in some ways, was actually quite simple in its essence. He was the theoretician and she the popularizer; he charted the course and she drummed up the support; he was the brains and she the heart. Perón could be a galvanizing speaker to a crowd but he was not especially comfortable or effective in face-to-face or skin-to-skin contact. This was where Evita was at her best, and also at her happiest. In short, there were an excellent team; he took care of diplomats, businessmen, and politicians while she looked after the source of their political power, her beloved "shirtless ones." It is also worth noting that their marriage seems to have been characterized by complete fidelity, something not very common in that Latino culture.

As Perón's six-year term entered its second half, there were slight but unmistakable signs that his vision of a "new Argentina" was beginning to fray. The economy was not longer expanding so rapidly, meaning government resources were no longer adequate to meet every demand. Evita continued her social welfare activities, but her speeches seemed less benevolent and more strident in attacking her enemies, the number of which appeared to be growing. This slippage in image might be an inevitable outcome for a demagogue, or it might have been the early sign of serious illness.

Illness and Death

On a hot summer day in January 1950, Eva fainted during a public ceremony. She was hospitalized immediately and a few days later there was an official announcement that she had undergone an appendectomy. Later, one of her doctors claimed to have diagnosed cancer of the cervix (the opening of the uterus or womb) and advised surgery at the time, which he said she rejected vehemently. However, this claim is suspicious for several reasons. In the first place, none of the other doctors corroborated his story. Secondly, he did not tell Perón, which would certainly be unusual. Finally, Eva seemed to recover fully following the appendectomy and remained well for a year or longer, a highly unlikely course for cervical cancer.

By early 1951, however, there were signs that the First Lady was not well. She appeared to have lost weight, seemed paler than before, and had swelling of the ankles. Weight loss is a common symptom of cancer; the cardinal symptom of cervical cancer is persistent vaginal bleeding which over time would lead to anemia and this would be evident as pallor; and swelling of the ankles and legs often occurs with advanced cervical cancer because of obstruction of the lymphatic vessels in the pelvis. Nevertheless, she continued her frenetic pace of activities and dismissed any suggestions of illness as rumors designed to discredit Perónism.

On August 23, 1951, Eva fainted again and at this point she finally consented to be hospitalized and evaluated. The diagnosis announced officially was anemia, but the doctors told her husband that she had advanced cervical cancer. Perón was stunned by this news, particularly since his first wife had died at an early age of this very same disease, and her death was a protracted and painful one. He ordered a search for a top cancer surgeon and the Argentine diplomatic staff contacted Dr. George T. Pack, a well-known and highly regarded surgeon at New York's Sloan-Kettering Institute for

Cancer and Allied Diseases. Pack agreed to consult on the case and he flew to Buenos Aires in late October to examine his patient under anesthesia and then again for the operation on November 6, 1951. Blood transfusions were given and Pack performed a radical hysterectomy, an operation involving removal of uterus as well extensive dissection of adjacent tissues to remove sites of spread. The cancer was advanced and Pack later said he was pessimistic about any possibility of cure.

Astonishingly, Evita was unaware that Pack was her surgeon, believing an Argentine surgeon did the operation. In fact, she never met Pack and he saw her only after she was anesthetized. Further, she was never told of the diagnosis, although she may well have guessed it. This kind of secrecy and what her priest later called "pious lies" seem shocking today, but at the time they were not all that unusual.

Election day—the first in Argentine history in which women voted—came while Evita was still in the hospital and photographs of her casting her ballot from her hospital bed were widely publicized. She returned to the Presidential palace and tried to plunge back into her work. She brushed off any suggestions that she limit her activities and, when her doctors proposed any kind of treatment, she would usually snap that she could not be deterred from her mission to help the people. She probably received some radiation therapy postoperatively, and may have also had some chemotherapy (which was just then coming into use), but the downhill nature of her course was evident to all. She continued to lose weight and was in constant pain. By Perón's inauguration on June 4, 1952, she was no longer able to stand and had to be propped up with a wooden frame and covered with a fur coat as she rode to the ceremony in an open car. Over the next several weeks, she had intermittent episodes where she was not lucid, and her weight sunk to 78 pounds. On Saturday evening, July 26, came the official announcement that the "Spiritual Leader of the Nation" (a title conferred shortly before by the Argentine Congress) had died.

Her death set in motion an incredible display of mourning. A 30-day mourning period was proclaimed and business closed and all official functions ceased for several days. Every city in the country draped its light posts and flagpoles in black. Over two million people filed past her bier, many of them throwing themselves on her glass-covered casket. The Army set up kitchens to feed the throngs, lined up four abreast over 20 blocks. Reportedly, 16 mourners were crushed to death by the crowds and 4000 were hospitalized with injuries. The food workers' union cabled Pope Pius XII, asking, "in the name of 160,000 members that Your Holiness initiate the process of canonization of Eva Perón," a request the Vatican declined diplomatically.

It all went on for two weeks with no end in sight, when the government finally called a halt. The body was removed to a suite of rooms in the labor confederation building, under the supervision of Dr. Pedro Ara, Spanish cultural attaché in Buenos Aires and master embalmer. Ara had actually begun the embalming immediately after Eva's death, working all night to prepare the corpse for its initial public display. He now had the opportunity to continue his complicated process, at a more leisurely pace, of making something to last forever. Perón planned a huge memorial building with the centerpiece being Eva's corpse on permanent display, much as the Soviets had done with Lenin or the Chinese Communists would later do with Mao Tse-tung.

As Ara carried out his work, weeks stretched into months and months into years. The memorial building never got past the planning stage because Perónism got into trouble. The economy stagnated, partly because of two consecutive bad harvests, and the coalition of the Army, the workers, and the church—bodies that actually had little in common—began to fall apart. As there was more dissent, government forces became more repressive in dealing with it. How much Evita's absence influenced these problems is uncertain, but it surely did not help. Finally, on September 20, 1955, a little more than three years after her death, Perón was forced out of office and left the country to exile in Paraguay and later in Spain. He was replaced by a series of military dictatorships and the anti-Perónists now in power moved quickly to wipe out all trace of the hated one and especially his wife. Monuments were destroyed, names on buildings were removed or changed, and former supporters were purged, deported, and in some instances executed.

At this point, the tale ceases being simply bizarre and becomes unimaginable. The anti-Perónists did everything they could to wipe out the memory of Juan and Eva, but they could not decide what to do with the embalmed corpse on the third floor of a government building. Committees and other units of the government met over many months, trying to decide how to deal with this hated symbol. It was as though, even in death, she wielded some magical power over them. Ultimately, the body was moved to a military installation and then turned over to an Italian priest, who took it and disappeared. Six weeks later, the priest reappeared and gave the President, Pedro Aramburu, a sealed envelope that presumably contained information about what had happened to the body. The President did not open the envelope, but rather gave it to his lawyer with instructions that on his death it be given to the then-President to do with as he wished.

Fifteen years passed, and the Evita legend persisted and in some ways even grew stronger. In the late 1960s, civil unrest was rife in Argentina, as it was in much of the Western World, and Perónism had been re-discovered and embraced by a radical left wing group. On May 29, 1970, former President Aramburu, now living in retirement, was kidnapped by guerrillas. He was interrogated about his administration and he answered the questions put to him, even though some incriminated him. However, when asked about the location of Eva Perón's body, he responded—truthfully—that he did not know. He was threatened with execution and, when he still could not answer, the threat was carried out. With his death, his lawyer delivered the letter to the current President, as instructed, and it was found to contain only the names of a priest (who had since died) and a cemetery in Milan, Italy.

Two representatives of the Argentine government traveled *in cognito* to Milan and searched the records of the named cemetery, looking particularly for burials in 1955 or 1956. One record caught their eye. It involved a middle-aged woman allegedly born in Italy who had immigrated to Argentina and on her death there her body was returned for burial in her native land. One of the officials, disguised and carrying false identification as the dead woman's brother, then secured a permit from the authorities to exhume the body. On September 2, 1971, the coffin was disinterred, loaded in a truck and taken across several borders into Spain, to a villa in a suburb of Madrid when Perón now lived in exile with his third wife. Opened in the presence of the embalmer, Dr. Ara, who had been called from retirement in Madrid, the coffin contained the near-perfectly preserved body of Eva Perón.

About this time, Perónism began to regain respectability in Argentina, culminating in Perón being called back in triumph in 1973. Curiously, he left Eva's corpse behind when he returned, but when he died (of natural causes) a year later and was succeeded by his wife Isabel, she arranged for it to come home to Argentina. Isabel planned a pantheon to house the two Peróns under the inscription, "Linked in glory, we watch over the destiny of our Fatherland. Let no man use our memories to divide Argentina." However, the ever-shifting tides of Argentine politics shifted once again, and the plans for the elaborate building died. Finally, closure came when the then-government quietly turned the coffin and its contents over to Eva's mother and sisters and, in the early morning hours of October 22, 1976, Maria Eva Duarte de Perón finally came to rest in the Recoleta Cemetery in the heart of Buenos Aires. This burial ground is an elaborate jumble of opulent, mansion-like mausoleums where the great and near great of Argentina are interred. One of the more modest burial vaults is a black marble crypt identified as "Familia Duarte." There are no signs or other directions to it and only a small plaque identifies its most famous resident. Regardless, 50 and more years after her Eva Perón's death, it is easy to locate by following the constant stream of pilgrims.

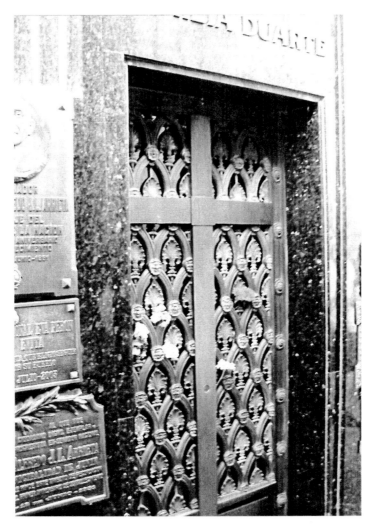

Figure 10.2 Duarte mausoleum, Recoleta Cemetery, Buenos Aires
(With permission from Pitkin RM *ACOG Clinical Review* 2004; 6: 11-6)

Medical Perspectives

The cervix, a cylindrical structure that forms the lower part of the uterus or
womb, contains a small canal leading into the uterine cavity and through this
canal menstrual discharge escapes, sperm ascend in their search for an egg to
fertilize and, after the canal is dilated substantially, a baby is born. The cervix
projects into the vagina and therefore can easily be seen and felt during a
gynecologic examination. Microscopically, the tissue covering the cervix
looks similar to the skin, being composed of 8-12 layers of flat, pavement-

like cells. These cells sometimes lose the normal mechanism that controls their growth and when this happens they begin to grow wildly, invading deeper tissues and spreading to other areas of the body, in the condition known as cancer of the cervix.

Exactly what causes cells to undergo malignant degeneration (i.e., become cancerous) is one of medicine's great mysteries, but in the case of cervical cancer, much has been learned by paying attention to the characteristics of women who develop the disease. An association with sexual activity has long been recognized. Cervical cancer, for practical purposes, does not occur in women with lifelong celibacy (such as nuns) and, moreover, its risk seems to increase with early onset of sexual activity and number of life-time sexual partners. All of these associations suggest some sexually trans-mitted factor and evidence accumulating over the past decade or so has identified this factor as the human papillomavirus (HPV). There are dozens of different types of HPV and only a few of them carry cancer risk. Women exposed to these high-risk forms of the virus apparently incorpo-rate its DNA into the genetic structure of their own cervical cells where, often after a long latent phase, it may cause the cells to turn malignant. Evidence of previous HPV infection can be found in nearly all cases of can-cer of the cervix. However, not all women with evidence of prior HPV infection develop cervical cancer, so there must be other modifying influ-ences. Among the characteristics that appear to modify risk are smoking (increased) and race (increased in black and Hispanic, decreased in Asian and white)

Cervical cancer has two distinct phases and it is essential to separate them in order to understand the clinical aspects of the disease. The two phases are best termed *preinvasive* and *invasive* and they need to be distinguished because they differ in so many ways. The preinvasive phase (that doctors often call cervical intraepithelial neoplasia or dysplasia) is when, on micro-scopic examination of a small piece of tissue, the cells in the 8-12 layers com-prising the surface underlineindividually begin to assume a cancer-like appearance. However, all the abnormal-appearing cells still remain within that superficial layer and none invade beneath it, into the deeper structures. There are no symptoms nor are there any changes recognizable to the naked eye. Thus, the woman with the condition and the doctor who examines her would have no indication that everything is not entirely normal. The preinvasive phase can persist unchanged for a long time, sometimes many years, and there can probably be spontaneous reversion to normal in some cases during this peri-od. Treatment during this time, consisting usually of relatively simple meas-ures directed at removing or destroying the small area of abnormal tissue, is highly effective. The cure rate is nearly 100%, although affected individuals have some risk of the condition coming back later, so periodic follow-up examinations are necessary.

George Papanicolaou, a Greek-American anatomist, made one of the most important discoveries in the history of cancer control in the 1940s. He was trying to time the reproductive cycle, using microscopic characteristics of cells collected from the vagina, when he noted that sometimes there were individual cells that looked as though they might be cancerous. He reasoned that these had probably been shed from the cervix, since cancer of the vagina is extremely rare, and thus was born a screening test for the preinvasive stage of cervical cancer that has saved countless women's lives over the past 50 years. It is simple, requiring only a gentle scrape of the cervix during the examination. Cells removed by this scraping are smeared on a slide and then taken to a laboratory where the slide is stained in preparation for microscopic examination. The test is especially suitable for use in women without symptoms or abnormal physical findings, who would otherwise be dismissed as normal. However, in these women the presence of cervical cells seen microscopically to be not normal can identify the need for more detailed examination and, ultimately, treatment. George Papanicolaou achieved a well-deserved measure of immortality in having the test designated by a shortened version of his name—the Pap smear or Pap test.

Beginning in the 1950s, in the United States and virtually all other industrialized countries, massive public educational programs were mounted to educate women about this approach and screening programs based on the Pap smear were set up. Over many years, a standardized protocol for using this approach and interpreting the results has evolved. It is important to understand that the Pap smear is a screening device and, while it may lead to a diagnosis, it cannot make a diagnosis by itself. If microscopic examination shows only normal cells, and especially if previous smears were always normal, the woman can be reasonably reassured that she is at no danger of developing cervical cancer for at least a year or so. If, on the other hand, cells that appear abnormal or suspicious are seen, then further study is needed. Sometimes the abnormality is so mild that the test need only be repeated in a few weeks. However, it the picture is frankly abnormal the first time or persistently suspicious, the next step is to excise a small bit of cervical tissue for processing and microscopic examination. This can often be aided by using a magnifying instrument called a colposcope to identify areas from which to take the tissue (remembering that there are typically no cervical abnormalities to be seen with the naked eye when the disease is preinvasive). If the diagnosis of preinvasive cervical cancer is made, it can be treated by the simple means mentioned previously, with the expectation of nearly 100% cure.

The Pap test is not perfect. Fairly often, it is reported as suspicious or even abnormal and a subsequent thorough investigation reveals that everything is normal. Sometimes, a Pap smear misses a significant abnormality; this is the reason annual tests are advised. The current recommendation regarding frequency of testing in healthy women, endorsed by the American College of Obstetricians and Gynecologists, the American Medical Association, the American Cancer Society, and the National Cancer Institute of the National Institutes of Health, is as follows:

> *All sexually active women or those who have been sexually active should, beginning at age 18, have yearly Pap smears and pelvic examinations; after three or more consecutive negative smears, Pap smears may be performed less frequently at the discretion of the physician.*

As noted, the preinvasive phase may last a long time and there may even be regression to normal; however, once the disease becomes invasive (i.e., once the abnormal cells, usually aggregated together, invade deeper tissues of the cervix) the situation changes. Quite quickly, vaginal bleeding (or occasionally non-bloody discharge) develops and there is an area of abnormality on the cervix evident on physical examination. The malignant tumor also tends to spread, typically sideways toward the pelvic wall and the lymph nodes lying alongside the large arteries and veins in the pelvis, but occasionally toward the bladder in the front or the rectum behind, and rarely to distant sites such as the lung or liver. In contrast to the preinvasive phase, there is some urgency once invasion has occurred since progression to advanced disease can take place over a few months. Also in contrast to the preinvasive phase, the treatment required depends on the apparent extent of the disease, but it is always major and carries some risk of complications.

One option for treatment is surgery, specifically radical hysterectomy. The term hysterectomy means removal of the uterus and most hysterectomies are the simple variety in which only the uterus is taken out (sometimes along with the tubes and ovaries). The radical hysterectomy is a more major operation in which, in addition to the uterus, the adjacent tissue extending to the pelvic sidewall is removed as well. Additionally, the lymph nodes to which the uterus drains are excised. The operation is time-consuming and tedious and must be done with great care because the large pelvic arteries and veins and the ureter (the tube by which urine gets from the kidneys to the bladder) are in close proximity.

The other treatment option is radiation therapy, typically given in two complementary ways. The first is a radioactive substance such as radium or cesium placed against the cervix where it is left for two or three days; this treats mainly the local area of the cervix. The second involves external treatments given with a machine, usually once per day for six weeks or so; this treats primarily the routes of spread in the pelvis. Originally, external therapy given with x-ray machines, but now higher energy sources such as the linear accelerator are used.

Either radical surgery or radiotherapy can be used in cases in which the malignancy seems on physical examination to be confined to the cervix (called stage I). Nowadays, some 85-90% of such women can expect to be alive and without evidence of disease 5 years after treatment, regardless of whether it was surgery or radiotherapy. Complications can occur with either and their frequency seems about the same. Complications from surgery tend to occur early whereas adverse effects from radiation may be late. Most gynecologic cancer specialists prefer surgery to treat stage I cases as long as the woman's age, body habitus, and general state of health make her a reasonably good surgical candidate; for other stage I cases and all women with higher stages, radiation therapy is generally favored.

The outcome of treatment depends more than anything else on the extent of disease. As noted, when it seems to be confined to the cervix, the 5-year survival rate is typically 85-90%. Modern radiation therapy gives rates in the range of 65-70% when tumor has spread toward the pelvic wall but has not reached it (stage II) and 40-45% when tumor has extended to the pelvic wall (stage III). In stage IV cases, in which the cancer has extended into the bladder or the rectum or spread outside the pelvis, the outlook is poorer and only 10-20% of treated women will be alive and apparently well in 5 years.

Statistics for cancer of the cervix, kept only for the invasive variety, have demonstrated remarkable improvements in outcome as a result of Pap smear screening programs. In the United States, for example, new cases of invasive cervical cancer annually fell by 76% (from 32.6 to 7.9 per 100,000) over the period of 1950 to 1990, and death rates from the disease declined similarly. These dramatic figures are due almost entirely to case finding and treatment of preinvasive stages, thereby preventing the development of invasive disease. In fact, cervical cancer probably constitutes the prime example of cancer control by a combination of public and professional education, leading to diagnosis and treatment at an early stage when cure is virtually assured. In contrast, outcomes with other cancers in women have fallen little or none and one has increased alarmingly. The graph below illustrates death rates (number of deaths per 100,000 women) for cervical and lung cancers in U. S. women over the last half of the 20th century, showing that deaths due to the former fell by two-thirds while those caused by lung cancer increased more than six-fold; (for comparison, breast and colon cancer mortality rates in women stayed relatively constant, at 25-33 and 17-22, respectively, over the same period).

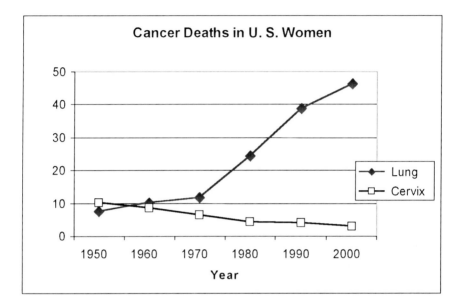

The encouraging statistics for cervical cancer apply throughout the developed world, but importantly they are limited to those countries having the resources for the public educational program and professional skills and equipment necessary. Areas of the world in which resources are so limited that professional manpower, clinical facilities and equipment, and public education simply do not exist have shown little if any improvement in either frequency or outcome of cancer of the cervix. Thus, while cervical cancer has fallen from the third or fourth to the eighth or tenth most common cause of cancer death in U.S. women, in many areas of the developing world, it ranks second only to breast cancer in this regard. Even in developed countries that have experienced phenomenal improvement, the disease has not disappeared entirely. The American Cancer Society estimates there were 12,000 new cases of invasive cervical cancer and 4000 deaths in the United States in 2000.

In 2006, after extensive research, a vaccine against four HPV strains responsible for most cases of cervical cancer, was released. Recommended for administration to girls before sexual activity is initiated, the vaccine is projected to prevent at least 70% of cases of cancer of the cervix. As with Pap smear screening, however, cost considerations limit this new technology to the developed world.

What do all these development and advances in cervical cancer mean with respect to Eva Perón and her illness? First of all, she fit the profile of risk factors, specifically early sexual exposure and multiple sexual partners. As noted previously, Juan Perón's first wife died of cervical cancer, raising the intriguing speculation that Perón himself might have been the source of a particularly virulent HPV. In any case, had Evita been born 50 (or perhaps even 20) years later than she was, in the well-developed medical environment of Buenos Aires she would surely have undergone Pap smear screening that would have led to diagnosis and treatment, and she would not have died of cervical cancer. As it was, she stands as a prominent historical figure reminding us of this scourge of womankind, a scourge whose elimination seems elusively just beyond our grasp.

SOURCES

Barnes J. *Evita First Lady: A Biography of Eva Perón*. Grove Press, Inc. New York. 1978.

Fraser N, Navarro M. *Evita*. W. W. Norton & Company. New York 1980. (Reissued 1996).

Taylor JM *Eva Perón: The Myths of a Woman*. University of Chicago Press. Chicago 1979.

Peron E. *Evita: in my own Words*. Translated from Spanish by Laura Dail. The New Press. New York. 1996.

Lerner BH. The illness and death of Eva Perón: cancer, politics, and secrecy. *Lancet* 2000;355:1988-91.

www.cdc.gov.nchs/data/vsus/mort. Accessed December 20, 2008

www.cancer.org. Accessed February 25, 2008

CHAPTER 11

MARIO LANZA AND
ISCHEMIC HEART DISEASE

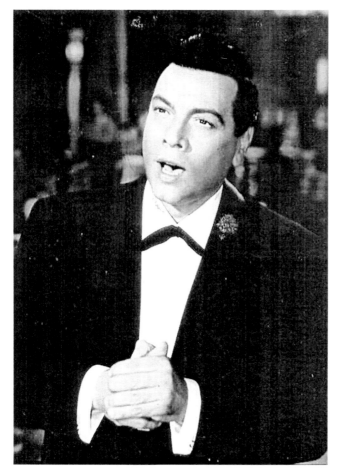

Figure 11.1 Mario Lanza (Courtesy of Bob Dolfi of Lanza Legend)

Mario Lanza, even though he did not follow the long and arduous training considered essential for an opera career, possessed a voice that stirred and excited many music lovers. He had an incredible range, reaching high notes effortlessly that other tenors could only dream about, and in the lower register his voice had almost a baritonal richness. His musicality and diction were perfect and, as added bonuses, he was handsome and had an engaging manner. He and everyone else assumed he was destined for a career in the world's finest opera houses, but instead he made his way in film and recording, leading some to deride him as simply a "movie singer." However, many of his detractors, on hearing him in person, acknowledged his enormous natural talent. His career lasted scarcely more than a decade before he died at 38 years of age, probably from ischemic heart disease, a premature death probably brought on by dietary excesses and cigarette smoking. Deaths due to this disease have declined by nearly half over the past quarter-century, but it remains the leading cause of death in the United States and other industrialized countries.

<u>Biography</u>

The story of Mario Lanza begins in the "Little Italy" area of South Philadelphia. To this day, the strong Italian influence is readily apparent, although it clearly has been diluted recently by immigrants from Southeast Asia. Around the turn of the century, the population consisted almost entirely of recent arrivals from Italy. One of them, Salvatore Lanza, had come in 1902 and was joined the next year by his wife and infant daughter, Maria. Another Little Italy resident was Antonio Cocozza who had enlisted in the army of his new country when it entered World War I and was wounded in battle, earning a citation for bravery along with a pension for a permanent disability.

In early 1920, the 26-year-old war hero married the attractive 16-year-old Maria and the couple joined her parents in their living quarters above the Lanza grocery store. On January 31, 1921, Maria gave birth to a boy, given the name of Alfred Arnold Cocozza. He was called Freddie and Freddie he would always be to the family, but the world would come to know him by the masculine form of his mother's name, a stage name he assumed at the beginning of his career.

Young Freddie, growing up in the tight-knit Italian community of South Philadelphia, was a popular kid, with an effervescent, charming personality and great personal warmth. His loved sports, especially baseball, football, and boxing, and he had better than average athletic ability. School was rather a different matter, for he was an indifferent student. But from the beginning, music was clearly his driving force. His mother had a good singing voice and his father was the kind of passionate devotee of opera found especially among Italians. Freddie grew up surrounded by his father's extensive record collection and very early he could be found listening to tenor arias repeatedly. By the age of ten he knew the plots and parts of 50 or more operas. He saw his first live opera at the age of 12 when his parents took him to a performance of *Aida*, and from that moment there was no doubt in his mind that opera would be his career.

His parents were skeptical initially about a musical career for their only child, but when they first heard him sing formally, they became convinced. They arranged for lessons—not voice lessons, for a 15 or 16-year-old boy is not mature enough for those rigors—but instruction in Italian and sight-reading music. Freddie did well in Italian but he had neither interest nor aptitude for sight-reading, a deficiency that would later hinder his career. By the time he was 18, he was ready to work on developing his voice, first with a local opera company and then with a private teacher. To cover the costs of private lessons, his parents took extra jobs. Freddie began to develop a local reputation, especially after Christmas morning 1940, when he sang *Ave Maria* at his neighborhood church. It was about this time that he adopted his stage name, Mario Lanza.

Mario's first big break came in early 1942 with an audition with Serge Koussevitzky, the great conductor of the Boston Symphony. On hearing the 21-year-old tenor sing the famous tenor aria from *I Pagliacci,* the maestro was enormously impressed and he invited Mario to the Berkshire Music Center in Tanglewood, Massachusetts on a full scholarship. The course of study there was rigorous and the conductors difficult and demanding, but Mario learned a number of different roles and got many performances under his belt. Tanglewood was widely recognized as the major proving ground for new musical talent and Mario's voice received favorable notice in several important publications; *Opera News* called him "a real find of the season" and one who "would have no difficulty one day being asked to join the Metropolitan Opera."

Then the rising career hit a snag. America had entered World War II and Mario Lanza, along with hundreds of thousands of other young men, received a letter from his local draft board that began "Greetings." He pled physical problems (poor vision in his left eye) and several advocates wrote letters telling what a tragedy it would be if his musical education were interrupted. But the draft board was unmoved, and in early 1943 the budding opera star was ordered to active duty. He did not enjoy his military career—not very many did—but it would be wrong to call the experience a hardship.

Quite early he was placed in a special unit touring the country entertaining troops, and later he found himself in the cast of a highly successful play that glorified the Army Air Corps and fueled the nation's patriotic fervor. If Mario did not gain much in the way of vocal training during his two-year military career (in January 1945, he was granted a medical discharge because of ear infections and postnasal drip), he certainly made a number of contacts and acquaintances that would prove useful later. One was Bert Hicks, a budding actor who introduced Mario to his sister, Betty. It was love at first sight and Mario and Betty were married soon after Mario's Army service ended.

The newlyweds settled in New York and Mario took up his singing career. Several jobs came his way, most notably a spot on a weekly radio program, *Great Moments in Music,* as a replacement for the noted tenor Jan Peerce who had previous commitments. Money was coming in, although not at the rate it was being spent it, for even early in his career Mario had already developed profligate ways. A chance meeting with Sam Weiler, who had become wealthy in real estate dealings and hotel management, provided a solution to Lanza's financial disarray. Weiler agreed to take over the singer's business management, paying off his accumulated debts and placing him on a monthly allowance, in return for a fixed percentage of his eventual income. Weiler had aspired to an operatic career himself, aspirations that were quietly shelved when he realized how limited his talent was compared to Lanza's, so he also became a mentor and artistic advisor as well as manager. It was a superb arrangement initially, but in later years it would lead to spectacular problems.

With Weiler's advice and encouragement, Mario began intensive study under Enrico Rosati, considered by many the world's greatest voice teacher. Rosati recognized immediately the incredible native talent of his new student, whose range extended two and a half octaves and whose innate musicality exceeded that of even his most illustrious previous pupils. Under Rosati, Lanza learned the diaphragmatic support, breath control, and facial muscle relaxation that would permit him to sing difficult passages for very long periods in an entirely natural way. Rosati permitted his pupil to sing an occasional concert but he insisted they be very limited in both number and length. Lanza performed in Toronto, Ottawa, St. Louis, and Chicago, all to rave notices from critics not noted for their generosity.

Despite Rosati's efforts to protect his star pupil from premature exploitation, by early 1947 his theatrical agency had booked a number of concerts involving the tenor. The idea was to put together several budding opera stars to tour the country, giving concerts to a public starved for culture by the recent war's austerity. The group, christened the Bel Canto Trio, was comprised of lyric soprano Frances Yeend and bass-baritone George London. The tour was a smashing success and Lanza was generally recognized as its star. It was also a time where he developed artistically. Coming off the period of intensive study with Rosati, he applied himself better than he ever would or could later and he continued to improve his techniques. He also learned from his colleagues, both dedicated artists, and from the accompanists. The tour provided reasonable income and it was also a time of personal happiness, for his adoring Betty usually accompanied him. He would always look back on the Bel Canto Trio as the best of times.

On the night of August 28, 1947, the crowd at the Hollywood Bowl numbered less than a fifth of the 20,000 capacity. The main performer was a 26-year-old tenor with a modest reputation and no tract record of ever having sung an opera professionally. He was there because the singer scheduled originally had cancelled. Yet when Mario Lanza began to sing—first a couple of duets and then arias by Verdi, Puccini, Donizetti, and Giordano—the audience was entranced. When he finished, they gave him a 12-minute ovation, one of the longest in bowl history. The Los Angeles press the next day was no less enthusiastic, with critics trying to outdo one another in superlatives. In the audience that night was movie mogul Louis B. Mayer who immediately signed Lanza to a seven-year contract. Mario insisted that the contract cover only six months each year, leaving him time to develop the operatic career that was his ultimate goal. The association with M-G-M, along with the recordings and personal appearances that flowed from it, would bring him worldwide superstar status and wealth beyond his wildest imagination, but it would also make him at the end more confused and insecure than he had ever been.

M-G-M assigned Joe Pasternak, a producer who had previously worked with serious musical artists, to introduce the new find to the making of movies. Pasternak was noted for making movies that offered a combination of "highbrow" and popular music and—most importantly—were successful commercially. He later said he thought it would take ten movies to make Mario Lanza a star, but actually it took only three. First came *That Midnight Kiss,* released in late 1949, and followed a year later by *The Toast of New Orleans,* with Kathryn Grayson co-starring in both. Each had a few operatic numbers, along with some lighter offerings such as those by Jerome Kern. Both films received positive, if not wildly enthusiastic, reviews and were successful commercially.

But the next film, *The Great Caruso,* a highly fictionalized story about the tenor generally regarded as the best ever, was a resounding success. The role was made for Mario Lanza, for Caruso was his idol, the person whose recordings he had listened to so intently as a child. It contained many operatic arias and duets and, when it was released on April 12, 1951, there was an avalanche of acclaim. Critics commented on the warmth and feeling of Lanza's singing, the thrill of his high notes contrasted with the softness and depth of the more tender portions, and the preciseness of his diction. Audiences all over the world simply loved it. *Time* magazine put Mario on its cover on August 6, 1951, calling him "the first operatic tenor in history to become a full-blown Hollywood star." The film's success led to surging public interest in opera generally.

Perhaps Mario Lanza as a movie star should not be any surprise, for with his matinee-idol good looks and his effervescent, engaging personality, he seemed made for the silver screen. But he and everyone else assumed all along that he would be an opera star. When asked about it, he would say that he was still young and there was plenty of time for opera. But as the years passed and his fame and wealth grew, while he still claimed he would eventually get to it, it became clearer and clearer that he was in no position to embark on the austere developmental program an opera singer first needs to complete. He could sing operatic arias, duets, and ensembles, as he did no fewer than 23 times in *The Great Caruso* and on countless other occasions on records, radio shows, and concerts. However, to actually perform an opera, at least at the highest level such as the Metropolitan or La Scala, required learning something in addition to the music, and this meant years of studying with demanding teachers and performing in second and third rank opera houses in Europe. With each step he took on the road to fame and fortune, this long and arduous preparation became less and less likely. Nevertheless, he clung to the idea of an operatic career until virtually the day he died.

The worlds of opera and movies are vastly different, and unqualified success in both is difficult if not impossible. The primary consideration in opera is artistic, whereas the driving force in movies is almost entirely financial. Further, people in opera regard movies, along with radio, television, and recording, as lesser endeavors because the performer has the option to do it over and over again until it is right, as opposed to "laying it on the line" once and for all the world to see. Moreover, sound engineering can compensate for weak volume and other vocal weaknesses in ways not available to the operatic performer. Lanza had some detractors who made exactly these points, but many of them recanted when they heard him sing live in concerts.

He did perform one opera professionally. It came very early in his movie career, during the six months he was free of commitments to MGM. He sang the role of Pinkerton in Puccini's *Madama Butterfly,* a production of the New Orleans Opera Association on April 8 and 10, 1948. But there would be no more. Perhaps that is the reason the naval uniform he wore in the part is displayed in the Mario Lanza museum in Philadelphia. Even if his performance record was minimal, he exerted a major effect in popularizing opera and bringing it to much of the public that would not otherwise have given it a second thought. He also inspired successive generations of opera singers; the three tenors, Pavarotti, Domingo, and Carreras, have each acknowledged the importance hearing Lanza was to the development of their careers. Even Elvis Presley once said that Mario Lanza had the strongest influence on his own singing style.

The huge success of *The Great Caruso* was followed by a triumphal concert tour, smashing record sales, and a rather mediocre movie, *Because You're Mine.* Soon, however, the glitter began to fade. Mario had great hopes for a new movie, *The Student Prince,* as an appropriate follow-up to *The Great Caruso.* It was an appealing story and the Sigmund Romberg score, while not exactly operatic, was reasonably close. Moreover, his co-star was the talented Ann Blyth, who had played opposite him as Caruso's wife in the earlier success. Unfortunately, the project kept getting delayed and when it finally got underway, disaster was just around the corner. The director criticized the star as over-emotional in an early scene. One thing led to another, and Mario walked off the set and demanded the director be replaced. Eventually, things were patched up and the work schedule moved to recording the musical numbers. Customarily in movies, the soundtrack is recorded in a studio and the singers then mouth the lyrics during the actual filming. Mario was well prepared for the recording sessions, which went smoothly and were completed in just two weeks. But when rehearsals began, trouble between star and director flared again, and this time there was no room for negotiation or compromise. After many months, during which the movie was in limbo, M-G-M sued Lanza for breach of contract. Again, there was much acrimony on both sides, until ultimately a deal was struck by which the studio would drop the suit in return for the right to use the already-recorded soundtrack with another actor. Eventually, the movie was made, with Edmund Purdom in the title role, mouthing the songs sung by Mario Lanza.

During the time of all the problems with *The Student Prince,* and quite likely contributing to them, another blow fell. Lanza learned that virtually all the money he had made in the last five years had been lost in a series of bad investments by his manager, Sam Weiler, and in addition he owed back taxes exceeding $250,000. It was difficult for Mario to believe that Weiler, his friend and mentor, had been so inept. There was a lawsuit and a counter suit, and when it was all settled, Lanza received a modest amount of cash and agreed to pay Weiler 5% of all future earnings.

The split with M-G-M and the breakup with Weiler took a heavy toll. The tenor's emotional stability began to show signs of cracking and he started drinking heavily. A television spectacular and a Las Vegas nightclub show, two new and different activities for Lanza, were tried in efforts to restore his failing career and replenish his depleted bank account. Both were fiascos. Because of a bad case of stage fright, on the television show he lip-synced earlier recordings, and the deception was obvious to everyone watching. He failed to even show up for the Las Vegas appearance; the official reason was a respiratory infection but he was upstairs in the hotel, too drunk to go on stage. About the only thing approaching a bright spot was one reasonably successful movie, *Serenade,* for Warner Brothers in 1956.

Mario had long been interested in visiting Italy, the land of his ancestors, and by early 1957 such a trip seemed more and more attractive. It would get him out of Hollywood and allow him a chance at a new start in Europe where he had a large and loyal following. He may have even still harbored thoughts of fulfilling his dreams of an operatic career, but everyone else knew this time had passed. Arrangements were made to rent an elaborate villa in an exclusive neighborhood of Rome, sufficient to accommodate Mario, his wife, their four children, and a number of servants. The entourage traveled by train from California to New York where, on May 17, 1957, they took ship for Naples. As the *Giulio Cesare* sailed out of New York harbor, Mario Lanza had no way of knowing that he was seeing his native land for the last time.

Illness and Death

The reception in Italy, where Mario Lanza was widely regarded as Caruso's successor, did much to restore the singer's confidence, at least temporarily. He began working almost immediately on a movie, *Seven Hills of Rome,* for which he would be paid $200,000 plus 30% of the gross. First, however, he had to enter a clinic for an intensive weight loss program, his weight having ballooned to 243 pounds. He lost 30 pounds in nine days and by the completion of filming was down to 169 pounds. His wildly fluctuating weight was by now a familiar pattern.

Concert tours were also arranged and, most importantly, he received an invitation to sing a Command Performance at the London Palladium in the presence of Queen Elizabeth II. Of course, he accepted this flattering invitation, but his preparations began ominously. He had great anxieties about losing his voice or forgetting his lyrics, and as a result he drank heavily and practiced only intermittently in the weeks preceding the performance, scheduled for November 17, 1957. Arriving at London's Victoria station, he was met by a cheering throng of admirers and in the press of the crowd the singer was actually injured slightly. Reaching his hotel, he began drinking and continued for several days. Then on the day before the performance he abruptly stopped, slept for some hours, and awakened seemingly in top condition. When he stepped before the lights and the audience of 2300, he was visibly nervous—not surprisingly, since he had not sung a live concert for seven years—but this passed and he gave an absolutely smashing performance. The critics, many of whom were skeptical beforehand, were wildly rapturous.

A European concert began auspiciously right after the New Year. However, he slipped and fell while in London, bruising his rib cage and injuring a leg. He continued with the scheduled concerts but, when he got to Germany several days later, he finally agreed to see a doctor. The doctor diagnosed phlebitis (inflammation of leg veins), high blood pressure, and an abscessed tooth, urging medical attention and complete rest. Mario sang one or two more concerts before finally giving in and canceling the rest of the tour. He entered the Valle Giulia, an expensive clinic near his home in Rome, under the care of Dr. Guido Moricca. After a few weeks, he left the clinic against his doctor's advice and, using a cane and with his leg in an elastic stocking, he flew to England to resume his concert tour. His phlebitis symptoms continued and he required injections for pain at nearly every stop. Also, there were frequent drinking bouts. Nevertheless, the crowds were large and responsive and the critics favorable, except for the occasional instances where performances were canceled. However, by the time he reached Hamburg in the middle of April, he could continue no longer. Although he did not know it at the time, Mario Lanza had sung his last concert.

Returning to Rome, he called his personal physician, Professor Giuseppe Stradone, who found him "in a precarious state of health," with an enlarged heart, evidence of abnormal liver function, and bronchitis, in addition to phlebitis. An electrocardiogram showed evidence of damage to the heart muscle due to insufficient coronary blood flow and this, coupled with an episode of chest pain on April 17, led to a diagnosis of a "minor heart attack." He was admitted to Valle Giulia and treated with diet and rest for several days. This seemed to rejuvenate him and he was able to make several recordings, notably a new stereophonic record of *The Student Prince*. However, his health clearly was failing.

In late August he was hospitalized with what was announced as "double pneumonia" but he quite likely had had another acute coronary occlusion. Electrocardiograms in August and September were interpreted as showing "hypertensive heart disease with arteriosclerosis." Plans were floated for another movie, but he was grossly overweight at 253 pounds and he therefore entered Valle Giulia for rest and weight reduction. It was considered an elective admission when he was driven to the clinic on September 25, to occupy his usual suite of rooms in the building's most secluded wing. Over the next two weeks, he did rest and he even sang several operatic arias for the staff. Then, on Wednesday morning, October 8, 1959, just a couple of days before his discharge was planned and immediately after his doctor had examined him, the singer was found lying on a divan, slumped over and non-responsive. All attempts to resuscitate him were unsuccessful.

As befitting a worldwide celebrity, Mario Lanza had three separate funeral services, each in a different area of the world. His body was taken to his home of the last two years, the Villa Badoglio, where it lay in state for two days. Then there was a service at the Immaculate Heart of Mary Cathedral in Piazza Euclide, with thousands lining the route, where the Roman Polyphonic Choir sang and Lanza's recording of *Ave Maria* was played. Then the body, along with the family, was flown to Philadelphia, where 15,000 people filed past the bier at Leonetti funeral home, and the

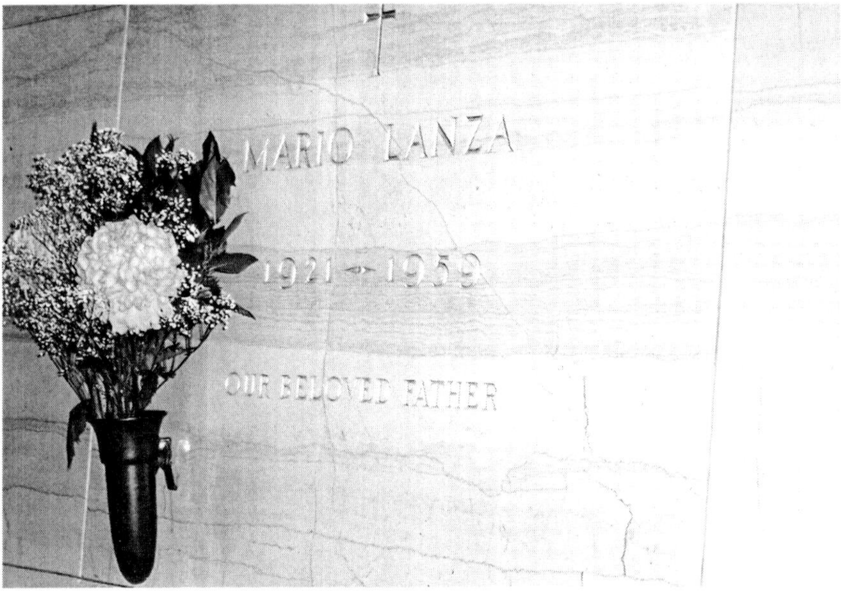

Figure 11.2 Lanza tomb,
Mausoleum of Holy Cross Cemetery, Culver City, CA

following day a requiem mass was celebrated at Saint Mary Magdalen di Pazzi where Mario had served as an altar boy and had sung the Bach-Gounod *Ave Maria* nearly 20 years earlier. Finally, the body was flown to its final destination, the place of Mario Lanza's greatest triumphs. There was a funeral mass at Blessed Sacrament Church in Hollywood, attended by many film luminaries, and then he came to rest in the hilltop mausoleum of Holy Cross Cemetery in Culver City, in a choice crypt just to the right of the chapel's altar. Mario Lanza's short but spectacular journey though life was over. Betty would join him within a year.

The magnificent voice may have been silenced in one way, but it lived on in the recordings and films that became his legacy, a legacy that has proved to be especially enduring. Mario Lanza societies and fan clubs continue to flourish around the world. There is a Mario Lanza museum and the Mario Lanza Institute in his native Philadelphia. The Institute, founded in 1964, sponsors a gala affair annually, at which it awards scholarships to promising young singers. A newsletter, *The Lanza Legend,* is published regularly and there is a web site (www.lanzalegend.com), both through the efforts of Bob Dolfi, a long time family friend, and Damon Lanza, Mario's elder son.

The cause of Lanza's death is not known with certainty. No autopsy was done but the consensus opinion, both at the time and subsequently, was that he died from an acute coronary occlusion. This diagnosis is, by all odds, the most likely. The clinical course is certainly consistent with an acute cardiac event, he was known to have coronary artery disease, and he had probably experienced at least two previous coronary episodes. There was also a possibility that he died from a pulmonary embolus, a blood clot from a leg vein that broke off and went to the lungs. His terminal course is certainly consistent with pulmonary embolus and he had suffered from phlebitis in the last weeks of his life. From time to time, more fanciful causes have been suggested. Probably the most absurd of these is the claim that he was murdered by the Mafia in retribution for failure to appear at a concert arranged by a Mafia kingpin. The final word on cause of death should be provided by his son, Damon Lanza, and Bob Dolfi, who went to Italy in 1998 and interviewed all the principals available. Their conclusion was unambiguous: Mario Lanza died of a heart attack due to extensive coronary heart disease.

Medical Perspectives

The heart, the most vital of the body's vital organs, is composed almost entirely of muscle and it contracts regularly, once each second or oftener, throughout an individual's life. When the heart ceases contracting or the contractions become ineffective, death ensues within a very few minutes. Blood flow to the heart, essential to supply oxygen and other nutrients and to remove waste products, comes through the right and left coronary arteries, each of which divides into several branches. Adequate blood flow is critical to heart function and any interference with it has serious and often fatal consequences.

As part of the aging process, coronary arteries tend to develop two types of changes collectively called arteriosclerosis. The first is a hardening and loss of elasticity of the arterial wall, so that its ability to dilate at times of need for increased flow (e.g., during physical exercise or excitement) is limited. The second (also called atherosclerosis) is the deposition of small areas of fatty substances, called plaques, at various places in the lining of the arteries. These plaques effectively narrow the diameter of the affected vessel, further limiting the volume of blood that can be pumped through the vessel in a given time. Moreover, blood flowing through the vessel can form a clot on a plaque, totally occluding the vessel and shutting off blood flow beyond. This acute occlusion of a coronary artery, commonly called a "heart attack," effectively shuts off the oxygen supply to the heart muscle beyond it or it can cause an erratic heart rhythm, either of which may be fatal.

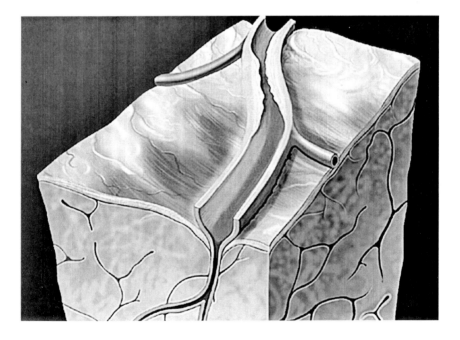

Figure 11.3 Drawing of coronary artery with arteriosclerotic narrowing
(Patrick J. Lynch © 2006)

Diseases of the heart represent the most common cause of death and disability in contemporary Western society, and the most frequent type of this category of disease is coronary arteriosclerosis. Also known as ischemic heart disease (i.e., heart disease due to ischemia or inadequate blood flow), this is the disease of the 20th century, for, while it was known earlier, its frequency has increased progressively during the last 75 years or so. In 1901, for example, all types of heart disease together ranked third (behind pneumonia and tuberculosis) as causes of death in Americans. However, heart disease quickly moved into first place and the ischemic type came to constitute at least two-thirds of all cases of heart disease. In the early 1950s, autopsies of soldiers killed in the Korean War demonstrated an unexpectedly high incidence of coronary artery disease among young and presumably healthy males. This was followed by an increase in clinical disease and in death rates, most alarmingly in younger and younger age groups, and led to a search for explanations and for effective means of prevention and treatment.

The number of deaths attributed to ischemic heart disease, after a progressive increase throughout most of this century, began to slow about 20 or 25 years ago and since then has decreased substantially. Between 1980 and 2000 in the United States, the age-adjusted mortality due to this diagnosis essentially halved, from 543 to 266 deaths per 100,000 population among men and from 263 to 134 deaths per 100,000 population among women. The cause of this beneficial trend is not known with certainty. Recent evidence suggests that about half can be attributed to improvements in medical treatment (including surgery of coronary disease) and about half to lowered risk factors (cholesterol lowering, hypertension control, smoking decrease, and more physical activity). In spite of this decline in mortality, ischemic heart disease is still the number one killer and it remains the most pressing public health problem in developed societies.

Five major risk factors for ischemic heart disease have been identified: high blood pressure, diabetes, high blood cholesterol levels, excessive body weight, and smoking. High blood pressure is a factor because, when the heart muscle is required to pump against increased pressure, it grows in much the same way a body builder's muscles enlarge with weight lifting. However, as the heart muscle increases in size, there is not a concomitant increase in coronary vessel number or size, so the blood supply can become relatively inadequate. In the case of diabetes, there is something about the metabolic derangements accompanying that disease, particularly when it is not well controlled, that predispose to accelerated development of hardening of arteries generally. Coronary arteries are usually involved, making ischemic heart disease a frequent complication in people with diabetes. Another fairly common site is the arteries of the lower extremity and individuals with long-standing diabetes sometimes must undergo amputation of a foot or leg.

Cholesterol, a fatty substance in food and also made by the body from other fats, can be elevated in blood because of either excessive dietary intake or an hereditary metabolic condition, or a combination of the two. The nutritional cause has received much emphasis, as the pervasive increase in dietary fats of animal origin during the 20th century paralleled the increase in ischemic heart disease in most cultures. Intensive educational programs mounted over the last decade or two have emphasized the importance of limited intake of cholesterol and saturated fats (which the body readily turns into cholesterol). Drugs that lower cholesterol, by interfering with its manufacture by the body, have been used widely since their introduction about 15 years ago and at present the most widely prescribed drug in the United States is one such agent. There is reasonably good evidence that cholesterol-lowering drugs are effective in preventing heart attacks due to acute coronary artery occlusion.

Excessive body weight increases risk of heart disease by at least two mechanisms: the excessive fat increases the work of the heart in pumping blood through it and the additional fat tends to raise the blood cholesterol level and blood pressure. Body weight of Americans has been increasing progressively over the past century, reflecting high intake of calorie-dense foods and diminished physical exercise. For the first time in human history, at least in industrialized societies, virtually all have ready access to food and freedom from the need for demanding physical work. Thus, what many have termed the "obesity epidemic" is a major public health concern in America today.

Rather than considering simply body weight, the modern diagnostic approach uses body mass index (BMI), a calculation that takes into account height as well as weight. The calculation is somewhat complicated but tables and automated methods are readily available (e.g., www.nchs.gov.org). The normal range for BMI is 18-24.9; values of 25-29.9 are considered overweight and those of 30 or more are termed obese. The most recent data indicate that among Americans aged 20-39 years, more than half have BMIs of 25 or more and a quarter have BMIs of 30 or more; of those aged 40 or more, the figures are even more alarming, 70% and 33%, respectively. It now appears that obesity has replaced tobacco has the number one modifiable behavioral factor causing death.

Finally, smoking is clearly responsible for a substantial portion of the increase in ischemic heart disease during the past century. Cigarette smoking became popular in the early 1900s, but the awareness of its adverse health effects did not come until later. The first major alarm came with the U. S. Surgeon General's report of 1964, with its emphasis on the relationship between smoking and lung cancer. Only later was a connection with heart disease appreciated. The mechanism by which smoking leads to ischemic heart disease is not entirely clear, but in part it involves the tendency for blood clotting at the site of arterial plaques. Whatever the mechanism, cigarette smoking is now well recognized as associated with accelerated coronary artery disease. Extensive public health campaigns have shown some effect in reducing smoking rates, which overall in the United States are now only about half of what they were a generation or two ago. However, success in smoking cessation efforts is far from complete (e.g., among young American women the rate continues to increase) and in much of the rest of the world, smoking shows little sign of diminishing.

Returning now to Mario Lanza, how do these well-recognized risk factors relate to his premature development of fatal ischemic heart disease? Of the five major risk factors, he lacked only diabetes. He smoked, as did many of his generation, and he definitely had high blood pressure. There is no specific information one way or the other with respect to his blood cholesterol level but his habitual diet was high in animal fats (e.g., it was not unusual for him to eat a dozen eggs for breakfast), so it would be astonishing if he did not have high blood cholesterol. His weight exhibited great fluctuation, as he would lose when necessary for a movie part or concert tour and then gain it all, and more, back. Overall, most of his life was spent at a higher-than-ideal weight. He himself regarded his optimal "singing" weight to be 200 pounds and, at his reported height of 5 feet 10 inches, this corresponds to a BMI of 28.7, well above the "overweight" threshold of 25. At times, by means of a "crash" diet and extensive exercise, he got down as low as 165 pounds, equivalent to a BMI of 23.9. However, on a number of occasions his weight ballooned to 260 pounds, a BMI of 37.3, well above the "obesity" threshold.

Not very much is known scientifically about the effects of "yo-yo" weight changes in which there is rapid and extensive loss, as result of severe dietary restriction and heavy exercise, and then weight is gained back just as rapidly, and so on through multiple cycles. Inevitably, weight lost this way would represent both fat and muscle, but when gained back the accumulation would almost certainly be all fat. Therefore, over several cycles the net effect must be central (i.e., abdominal) obesity, a well-recognized independent risk factor for ischemic heart disease.

Finally, there is the question of stress or tension and its effect on heart disease. It has long been believed that individuals in chronically stressful situations are at special risk to develop heart disease, but evidence to this point is lacking, perhaps because of the lack of any objective measure of stress. Lanza certainly had an artistic temperament and his life as a performer was filled with tension. What effect this had on is health is uncertain.

How would things have been different if Mario Lanza had been born 50 years later than he was, in 1971, so that he would be in his mid-thirties now? He certainly would have been exposed to information about the importance of a healthy diet and exercise and he would have been deluged with anti-smoking messages. Assuming these influenced him to exercise, maintain a healthy weight, and not smoke, he quite likely would not have developed ischemic heart disease at the early age he did. If his blood cholesterol were elevated, and even if it were normal in the face of demonstrable coronary artery disease, he would be treated with diet and cholesterol-lowering drugs. If he had evidence of actual heart disease, surgery would be a consideration, the approach depending on the severity. If there were limited involvement of only one or two vessels, the appropriate procedure might be angioplasty, in which a small catheter is passed through the groin artery and into the heart to dilate any area of obstruction, somewhat like the plumber who opens a clogged sewer pipe. With more extensive disease, a major operation called coronary artery bypass might be needed; in this case, the chest is opened and a vessel, usually a vein from the leg, is used to bypass an artery that has a number of obstructions.

In sum, then, had Mario Lanza lived 50 years later than he did, the strong probability—though far from a certainty—is that he would have avoided premature death due to ischemic heart disease. If he had, the world would have had more than just a few years to be thrilled by his magnificent voice.